"Dr. Bill Williams is doing great things in the name of dentistry and "The $10,000-a-Day Dentist" is his latest contribution—and one that I love to see. Passionate, intelligent people who give back to dentistry are my kind of people. Williams has a history of creating million-dollar and multi-million-dollar practices—and even better—he made it a life's work to catalog and record exactly how he did it every step of the way. He first shared his knowledge with "Marketing the Million Dollar Practice," and now with this book, he's proven that the sequel *can* be better than the original. This book doesn't beat around the bush or talk in circles like so many business books do these days; it's solid advice and real strategy from a doc who champions the union of business and dentistry."

Howard Farran, DDS, MBA
Founder of Dentaltown.com, and CEO and publisher of Dentaltown magazine
Best-selling author of "Uncomplicate Business: All It Takes Is People, Time, and Money"

"WOW... ARE YOU UP FOR AN 'out- of- the box' CHALLENGE?? Just read the Prologue, and you will NEVER do Dentistry the same again!! WHO WINS? The patient first! THEN, the Dentist and Staff, from this incredible ***'prophetic plan'*** for NOT ONLY increased productivity, but increased love for the 'ART FORM' we provide for our patients, utilizing 21ST Century Amazing Dentistry! Dr. Williams shares with Authenticity, Vulnerability and Amazing Experience!"

-Naomi Rhode
Phoenix AZ
CPAE Speaker Hall of Fame, Co-Founder SmartPractice

As always, Dr. Bill Williams is th
cheese - after it's been moved! The alw
expanding beyond self-imposed thoug
successfully conquered his own limitat

'Goliaths'. And now he shows us, once again, how we can do it, too. I say, Hurrah for champions like Dr. Bill Williams who mark the path, blaze the trail, and show us through his accomplished example how we can harden and polish our own metal - just as he has done.

- Lee Ostler DDS
Richland, WA
Past-President of American Academy for Oral Systemic Health (AAOSH)

Five Stars!!! I've had the honor and privilege to know Dr. Bill Williams as both a mentor and a friend. His new book, "The $10,000 A Day Dentist," is a solid pillar of knowledge that every dentist should read. In his book, Dr. Bill takes the reader on a journey through the eyes of Dr. Alex Middleton, the guide, the mentor, who has already been down the path and now leads others to their dreams and goals. Bill very well-describes what he calls "The Five Truths" and breaks down what it takes to become a "Decathlon Dentist." Bill Williams is a man of faith, integrity and character of the highest regard – as a guide and mentor, I can think of no one better to lead the charge for today's dentist.

-Dr. David Phelps, D.D.S.
Rockwall, TX
Owner and founder, Freedom Founders Mastermind Community

In *The $10,000 Dentist a Day*, Dr. Williams gives readers the tools to understand themselves, which is key to being the dentist you always wanted to be and leading a purpose-driven life. Easy to relate to, Dr. Williams teaches readers how to avoid bottlenecks and other obstacles to success. You'll finish the book with a better understanding of yourself, and how to take your future into your own hands.

-Tonya Lanthier, R.D.H.
Atlanta, GA
Founder DentalPost.net

Dr. Williams "The Decathalon Dentist" has devoted his life to clinical dental education and business mastery. In *The $10,000-a-Day Dentist,* Dr. Williams graciously shares insights into management systems which will help you run a more efficient and profitable dental practice. In this colorful and creative book, Dr. Williams teaches dentists how to free their time to be able to do more of what they love, dentistry. You will never tire of this entertaining and fantastic book. In the end, Dr. Williams reminds us that a well-designed day becomes not only the blueprint for success in dentistry, but also for life.

- Ann Marie Gorczyca, DMD, MPH, MS, Orthodontist,
Walnut Creek, CA
Author of the Books *It All Starts with Marketing, Beyond the Morning Huddle, and At Your Service*

Bill has been one of the most influential dentists in the US for many years. Now, he has given us a double helping of secret sauce! I am certain that the specialized knowledge gained from reading this book will 10X the momentum of your practice or DSO."

-Brady Frank DDS,
Medford, OR
Founder OsteoReady & Transition Time

I give "The $10,000 a Day Dentist" my highest endorsement. Everyone has a different measure of success and this book defines success on many high levels. Every super star, such as Michael Jordan, has a coach to sharpen their game. Oprah Winfrey herself speaks of having many mentors who helped pave the way to her success. I encourage you to join their proven path with Bill as he has the mentorship and wisdom you need to be successful in our world of dentistry!

Elijah Desmond, RDH
Delray Beach, FL
CEO Smiles at Sea

THE $10,000 A DAY DENTIST

50 Ways to Create a Highly Successful Practice

By
Dr. Bill Williams

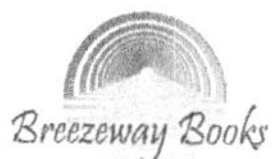

ISBN: 978-1-62550-513-2
978-1-62550-525-5

TABLE OF CONTENTS

FOREWORD

If you are a Dentist or Dental consultant, you will find new and valuable information (pearls) in Dr. Bill Williams' new book. It belongs on your bookshelf as a reference guide.

Dr. Bill has spent his career as a student, teacher, philosopher, author, and an example to all who strive to be the best they can be in their profession.

I have known Dr. Bill Williams for decades. He has always set and raised the high bar for excellence, not only in his work but also in his life balance.

He has seen the hard times as well as the very best of times in his career which gives him the unique opportunities to share both. In this book, he shares a thoughtful look at a complete career in Dentistry . . . turning obstacles to opportunities.

Importantly, he describes what you as a Dentist can do TODAY to further your success TODAY, with competence, confidence, and attitude of servitude for your patients.

This book has lasting meaning. Subsequent readings will reveal ideas not important in previous readings.

As a handbook for your career, this book deserves a permanent place on your book shelf.

Joe M Ellis DDS
Houston, TX

PROLOGUE

It was 8:30 AM on Friday, February 24, 2017, and Alex's big implant case that morning was already half an hour late. His morning huddle had gone off without a hitch, everyone was present and his business assistant had announced that he had just over eleven thousand dollars' worth of work scheduled for the day and there were no holes in the schedule to fill, which also meant no room for patients to be late starting their procedures. There was no way the day would end well.

At seven PM, Alex arrived home after a full day at the office. He handed the day sheet to his wife and said, "We did pretty well today." Besides seeing all of his regularly scheduled patients, even the late implant patient, he worked in three more implants on two patients and a three-unit bridge on another, finishing to finish the day's production at $22,000. He got his full lunch hour, ran errands, and worked on charts for the next week. The day was long, yes, but it had ended well, after all.

Alex was in his fourth decade as a dentist and had been instructing, lecturing, writing, and leading dentists for thirty-five of those years. In 2005, he made an amazing discovery and began implementing it into his practice. In 2011, he began sharing his discovery with other dentists. His is the story of the

$10,000-a-day dentist. Alex takes possibility to a new level as he helps dentists finish well, redefining dentistry with new constructs, like the Leap Frog strategy, the Gold Key List, the Dental Jungle, the 100-Day Challenge, Extra Dental Perception, the Swiss Army knife approach, the Dental Hot Seat, Free Time Anytime, 8@8, 3 in 3, and the Trump Effect.

Sound unbelievable or too good to be true? Read on, and you'll see how "chunking," or breaking a day down into smaller bites, can propel you. Alex has a goal of ten thousand a day and a plan to make it happen. Most days, he does 30-50% more than his goal. Welcome to Alex's world.

INTRODUCTION

Guide: "One that leads or directs another's way," according to *Webster's Dictionary*; "a person who advises others, especially in matters of behavior or belief," according to *The Oxford Dictionary*.

As dentists, we are touched by teachers, professors, mentors, authors, gurus, and guides. Conversely, we touch the lives of others as we take on those roles and begin influencing. As guides or mentors, we impact and alter the lives of those within our spheres of influence. In this book, you'll encounter Alex, a man who has influenced many people, not just dentists.

We go through life linearly, from career beginning to career end. But a mentor/guide like Alex may intersect with dentists in one of several phases of their careers. He may touch and moves on and perhaps return to give more direction.

"A mentor is someone who sees more talent and ability within you than you see in yourself and helps bring it out of you."

—Bob Proctor

Timing

Timing is everything, so dividing a dentist's career into four general quadrants is useful for study and commentary: (1)

Youthful, (2) Aware, (3) Peak performer, and (4) Mature. The first group is typically young, right out of dental college, new to practice, and perhaps associated with another dentist. They are lovingly called "baby docs." Everything is before them, and unfortunately, very little water has spilled over their dam. What they lack in experience, they make up for with enthusiasm and potential.

The second group may be five to ten years into practice and acutely aware of what they are doing. They consider themselves focused and experienced. They have developed social consciousness and awareness. These dentists feel that they are doing well enough to begin giving back to the community. This group can be called "the servant group."

Peak performers comprise the third segment on the career scale. With fifteen to twenty-five years in practice, they know the ropes, have hit their stride, have figured out many of the systems, and are well on their way to achieving success as dentists. They often believe they have reached the tops of their games. They operate at extremely high levels compared to the average dentist. Experience matters and these accomplished doctors have that plus a view of the end to motivate them to excel.

The fourth and final category is the mature dentist. For some, it's a time of fading away into the sunset, of blending into the woodwork. But for others, it's an accentuation of the peak performer phase, only faster and easier than ever. The mature dentist is typically between forty-five and sixty-five and actively planning his or her retirement, or at least thinking about it. The closer they come to realizing that Social Security will not be the answer, the more they try to figure out how to finish well.

A mentor/guide touching their career will greatly impact what they'll understand and the benefit of that interaction. It's true that one doesn't know what one doesn't know. Albert

Einstein once said, "The more I learn, the more I realize I don't know." If dentists could know everything they need to know in the beginning, it would be so easy, but they would not recognize the value if it came to them at the wrong time. The mindset and needs of a young dentist are diametrically opposite to that of a mature dentist. Matching mindset and methods with timing in a dentist's career is the most significant task of the mentor/guide.

THREE PATHWAYS

There are many highly acclaimed dentists who share how they found success. On any given day, one can find books by successful dentists and non-dentists that point to how to make it. Different paths can lead to the same destination. Each path may be unique yet reach common ground. Books like these are like treasure maps for finding the pot of gold. In this book, our guide Alex will be sharing fifty ways to be successful with the five doctors who come under his guidance, each of whom fall on one of three paths.

Path One: Mentor Leaders

At a crossroads, you have to choose which path to follow. How do you know which path to take? The path you select should make you comfortable. What fits best in your mind, in your psyche, in your paradigm? The answer depends on your personality and belief systems. Do you prefer to work with an authority figure or expert? Because they have proven themselves, you want to emulate them in your own practice. This type of guide speaks from personal experience. Path One gives you confidence that you are following a leader who will show you the correct way because they have lived and breathed the same situations and conditions. I've been blessed to have had Dr. Omer K. Reed, Dr. Ron McConnell, Dr. Charles Martin, Dr. Carl Misch, Pastor Katherine Ruonala, Arman Morin, Dave Dee, and many others function as personal mentors.

Path Two: Expert Guides

Perhaps you will choose to work with someone who will walk beside you and guide you to a place they have seen, where the proverbial pot of gold should be. This guide understands the signs of success and danger and will steer you towards better results and away from ruin and failure.

Dental consultants travel this path. We've hired many over the years: Kendrick Mercer, Quest Consultants, Arrowhead Consulting, Pentegra, Sunrise Dental Solutions, and Action Coaching. They have seen success and failure and know the terrain well. They may not have been in the same boat as you, but they have seen a lot of people who were. I've been fortunate to have many team members in our practice who went on to become top consultants in their fields, like Linda Drevenstedt, RDH; Jennifer McDonald; and Tonya Lanthier, RDH. Dentists need consultants and many are worth their weight in gold.

Path Three: Adventure Buddies

Your most successful learning style may be to find someone who will join the adventure and ride that street car named Desire with you in search of gold, wherever it may be. You're both looking for the same prize. You chose this method of growth because for you, the journey is as much the prize as the goal. I call this path the Buddy Path.

Many dentists want to adventure with another dentist. There is strength in combining resources with another dentist or group of dentists and working to the advantage of all.

Several times, I've been part of groups of dentists who came together to dig deeper into a specific subject, most notably the Atlanta Craniomandibular Society—twelve dentists from Georgia who met monthly for over twenty years, beginning in 1978. From that came more than nine international lecturers and clinicians in head, neck, and facial pain. Dr. Larry Tilley and I taught together for over ten years in TMJ Framework and the United States Dental Institute. Challenging each another, holding each another accountable, sharing in the learning process, and celebrating victories with likeminded others is a winning formula.

Later on, the Solstice Research Group was formed by nine strong dentists from across the USA and Canada to hone their skills in patient examination, diagnosis, and consultation. This group, whose beloved "papa-san" was Dr. Joe Ellis of Houston, Texas, stayed together for over a decade, meeting twice a year near the summer and winter solstices – hence, the name. You will hear from some of the members of the Solstice Group later in this book.

Enter the Forest

As you journey along your path, eventually you enter an enchanted forest of ideas. There will be many that stand out. These ideas (trees) may mean everything to you but nothing to the next person who reads these chapters (forest). These are the "Aha!" moments you seek, the hidden gems and diamonds just beneath your feet. They are the proverbial needles in haystacks that will tie so many loose ends together for you and your practice.

The ideas Alex shares may speak to you from these pages or come to you through your dreams and prayers once your mind has been activated by curiosity. Technology could connect you to Alex's message. Information is powerful, and once you are exposed to it you cannot ignore it. Alex will present his ideas to each dentist in the context of where they are in their careers. Timing is everything. You may recognize yourself in descriptions of our five dentists, who encounter our protagonist, Alex the Guide, as they journey along their individual paths.

THE $10,000 A DAY DENTIST

50 Ways to Create a
Highly Successful Practice

Chapter 1

PROVIDENCE

When you encounter something by chance that seems like it was meant to be, then it could be providence, your destiny.

Steve's Story

Steve sits at his breakfast table gazing past the frosted window pane at the falling snow. It's Friday. At least he's off. He can't imagine going in to work again on a Friday. He hasn't done that in years. While many of his friends are down in Florida, snow birds that they are, he's here in Minnesota, working four days a week. He's thinking, "What's the secret? Why can't I be where they are? Where did I go wrong?"

Fast forward seven years. Steve, on his forty-fourth Fourth of July as a practicing dentist, finally arrives at his own personal Freedom Day. As he places the hand piece in the rack for the last time and sits his longtime patient up in the dental chair, he smiles. He has drilled his last tooth and polished his last composite. Yes, he will miss the patients, but not the dentistry.

Steve is tired, but he is happy. His career is complete and he has finished well.

During the eight years between the winter of 2009 and now, Steve met with Alex, his mentor and guide, and learned about the art of leadership, management, communication, and marketing and gained tools to shape his own destiny. Alex shared with him how he had reduced his own number of work days over several years and had been able to maintain consistently productive days in the office. Alex taught him to build systems that allowed him to average over ten thousand dollars every day he came to work. Steve grew his already successful practice by 85% and was able to save more towards his retirement than he had originally thought possible.

When Steve was ready to transition the practice, he far outshone most of his colleagues. Steve added millions to his retirement nest egg from the buyout and bonuses he negotiated. After selling the practice, Steve stayed on, working three days a week for two years to ensure that the transition went well. He reduced his number of work days to just two days a week after the first two years. He enjoyed the opportunity to travel and still make a good income from his highly profitable days in the office. Cruising, camping, fishing, and golfing were more frequent as the years passed.

He purchased stock in the company, and by the time he cashed it in, it had quadrupled in value, further adding to his retirement. Alex was right; there was a pot of gold at the end of his dental rainbow, and he had found it!

Why?

Do you ever ask why? Are you often frustrated that you are not where you want to be in your life or practice? If you have ever found yourself pondering age-old questions but had only a blank wall staring back at you with no answers, then perhaps this book will open some doors for you and provide insights to get those answers you seek. Travel life's path with Alex as he shares five truths and a plethora of ways to achieve extraordinary success as a dentist.

"You see," said Alex, "there are four stages in a dentist's career and each has a set of truths to follow and methods to understand." When you have a guide, and when you know the path and the truth, then a course to success can be charted when the timing is right. "You can count on it."

The Guide: Dr. Alex Middleton

Born into a middle-class family with a strong work ethic in Atlanta, Georgia, Alex was a boomer baby, the son of fighters from the Greatest Generation and grandson to grandparents born before the twentieth century who weathered the Great Depression and came out stronger because of it. They were tested by the real world and succeeded in it.

A Solid Foundation

Alex grew up participating in Scouting. Integrity, honesty, God, and family were instilled in him early. Leadership and accomplishment were celebrated along the way. Scholarship and merit were rewarded, and goals were set and results achieved. College exposed him to alternatives and choices. Experience led to excess and a resetting of values. Tried and true values were substituted for thrills and troubles. Lessons were learned; growth occurred. Alex learned there were consequences.

Alex followed his own counsel when he became a professional dentist. At first, he tried to go it alone. When he sought out mentors, he realized that not seeking and heeding their advice had caused him pain.

"You see," said Alex, "I was pretty stubborn and thought I knew everything."

Lessons learned turned into lessons he would eventually teach. From the trials came a story and from the story came hope and more stories for thousands of dentists who would follow in the way of the guide.

Many of you may remember a TV hero named MacGyver, who played the role of a secret agent with almost infinite resourcefulness. He solved complex problems by making things out of ordinary objects utilizing his ever-present Swiss Army knife. MacGyver was like a fox: clever and intelligent. Dr. Alex Middleton was the dental version of Angus MacGyver. He taught the "Swiss Army knife" approach to dental practice growth.

Whenever Alex shared his story, dentists discovered a way to move beyond whatever held them back. Dr. Alex Middleton had "been there and done that." Most dentists could relate to him because he was a practicing dentist still in the trenches, wet-fingered and wet-gloved, not some fool in an ivory tower. He had succeeded and failed. But he had succeeded again in a much grander way, having learned invaluable lessons. Alex discovered how to turn stumbling blocks into stepping stones. He was a believer, inspired by the Word of God, who built his life and his second practice on a stronger foundation, incorporating the Word along the way.

As an Eagle Scout and member of the Order of the Arrow, Alex learned about the Eagle anointing. Like the eagle, Alex had the ability to shed the old and take on the new, just as eagles molt their old feathers to grow new ones so they can fly higher and farther.

"When it rains, all birds occupy shelter, but eagles avoid rain by flying above the clouds. Problem is common to all.

But ATTITUDE to solve the problem makes all the difference."

– Author unknown

This is a book about molting, then flying higher and further than you've ever gone. Taking on a new mindset enables you to navigate uncharted waters. Walk with us as we see how God's providence intersected the lives of five dentists and Alex, the guide. To whom do you most closely relate? Where are you on the timeline of your career?

The Mature Dentist: Dr. Steve Blake

You heard Steve's questions as he watched the snow from his breakfast table. Steve's high school classmates had begun to retire. Steve wanted to retire at age sixty-five. He was worried that he hadn't saved enough to live on. His practice grossed $800,000 a year as a solo dentist. He wanted to begin slowing down, yet was afraid it wouldn't happen easily.

Dr. Blake is fifty-eight and from Wayzata, Minnesota, looking to finish well. He clicked on Alex's Facebook post of a dental marketing book about building a million-dollar practice. He eventually joined Alex's group to be around like-minded, progressive dentists. When an open-minded, experienced dentist falls into a proven system for expanding and maximizing a dental practice, the truth is revealed: Your history is not your destiny.

The Peak Performer: Dr. Carley Matthews

Some people are attracted to challenges, to scaling higher heights than others. Mountaineers climb K2, the Matterhorn, and McKinley. Race car drivers compete in Daytona, Indy, or the 24 Hours of LeMans. Dentists enter residencies to become fellows and masters. They attend in-depth, comprehensive continuing education courses because peak learning experiences propel them toward their long-term goals.

Dr. Carley Matthews signed up for the first AAID Maxi-Course at the Medical College of Georgia and then later joined the Georgia AGD Mastertrack five-year program to complete her Mastership in the AGD. With twenty years in dentistry and a massive amount of experience, she was indeed a peak performer, one with gifted hands, an intellect to understand the nuances of many disciplines, and a likeable personality. In a nutshell, she had it all. Alex was in both programs and they became fast friends and colleagues. Providence, of course, and a destiny forever impacted.

The Servant: Dr. Edward Boyle

Dr. Edward Boyle googled the names of various countries and dental missions in Africa: Uganda, Tanzania, Chad, and Kenya. Ed wanted to do more than just local mission projects. He yearned to experience life in third world countries and to help make a difference for those with no real opportunity to have what he had. Dr. Boyle had been in practice ten years and was happy with his situation. He was a pillar of the community and well-respected among his peers. As a Rotarian whose motto is "Service above Self," he sought ways to use his dental skills for higher purposes.

As he continued to search, he found a picture of Kenya Medical Outreach's dental mission in the land of the Masai. Slowly, their story unfolded as Dr. Boyle followed the photo to the Kenya Medical Outreach website. There he found blogs about mission teams going back more than a decade, showing dentistry being done outdoors under shade trees, in primitive conditions, as lines of people looked on. Edward saw the beautiful faces of the Masai children and the hope in their parents' eyes as their children received medical and dental care. Edward sought more information on joining a team to Africa and found Dr. Alex Middleton.

After leading dental missions to Honduras and Kenya, Dr. Alex Middleton had gained a reputation for mission work. Dentists called to join his mission teams. Dr. Boyle was one such dentist. After they connected online, talking Rotary, travel, Africa, and missions, Edward knew his passion to serve would be fulfilled. Eventually, Ed traveled to Kenya and the Masai Mara with Alex several times as a mission team member. Providence indeed.

Baby Doc: Dr. Blair Bennett

The matchmaker works and watches, and watches and works. Alex first met Dr. Blair Bennett, a recent graduate of Emory University School of Dentistry, at the monthly session of the Atlanta Craniomandibular Society. Dr. Joe Konzelman, head of the Oral Medicine Department, introduced the two, explaining that Alex was one of the most forward-thinking dentists in the society and someone Blair should meet. Joe knew what he was doing. Blair was originally from Brooklyn, New York, and had moved to St. Petersburg, Florida, at the age of twelve and lived there until enrolling in Emory University in Atlanta. Blair's interest in joining Alex was based on Alex's expertise in TMJ and head, neck, and facial pain. Soon, Dr. Bennett was associated with Alex's practice. Providence it was, divine providence.

The Local Dentist: Dr. Jack Mudd

Alex walked into Dr. Mudd's office to introduce himself. Dr. Mudd just stood there, silent, like a stick. Such was the beginning of a strange coexistence. Dr. Jack Mudd lived and practiced in the same community as Alex and had been the only dentist in town for ten years. They were competitors, but it was a fast-growing community, and they were not likely to step on one another's toes. They attended the same dental study club. They had that in common, but little else.

Those five dentists, through providence, ran into Alex, the guide. Each was in a different place in his or her career. Each was in a different frame of mind, also. No two dentists are the same, but there are many similarities. You may see a bit of yourself in each of these.

As Alex got to know Drs. Bennett, Matthews, Mudd, Boyle, and Blake, they asked him questions and he asked them questions, but before one can know the answers, one must first know the Five Truths.

Chapter 2

SUCCESS

Success varies, but truth does not. One man's definition of success is another man's version of scarcity. For some, abundance is reached quite easily, yet for others it is a struggle that takes decades. That's why it's important and helpful to set a goal, to know what your winning score needs to be.

Where Does Success Come From?

Success comes from four things: (1) Perspiration, (2) Inspiration, (3) Family, and (4) the Silicon Sandbox. Sixty percent of all success comes from your work and your continuing education, what you learn after dental school in training classes, participation courses, and experience. It's the books, videos, online training, study clubs, and masterminds, plus the mentors and guides with whom you associate. It depends on you implementing what you have learned and putting knowledge into action. This work is the perspiration of successful people.

Twenty percent of success comes from inspiration, which comes from serious contemplation, dreams, meditation, and prayer. These elements are all important to success. One must have the proper mindset to achieve success, and listening to the voice of wisdom helps achieve success much faster than ignoring it. Dreams play a part in your success, too. At times, what comes to you in dreams is meaningful and has purpose. Prayer is always valuable, and God's word never returns to him void, so why not pray Jeremiah 29:11 (NIV): "'For I know the plans I have for you,' declares the LORD, 'plans to prosper you and not to harm you, plans to give you hope and a future.'"

Ten percent of success comes from your family. Morris Massey spoke extensively on three major periods during which values are developed: the Imprint Period, up to the age of seven; the Modeling Period, between the ages of eight and thirteen; and the Socialization Period, between thirteen and twenty-one. He says, "What you are is who you were when." I believe you can also have a second childhood and have an epiphany as a dentist if you join the right "family."

Ten percent of success can be achieved through what I call the silicon sandbox. You don't have to carry books, go to classes, remember facts, drive to the theater, or do time-wasting, heavy tasks any longer. It's all there in your hand with smart phones, iPads, and the like. You want to be on the right side of the digital divide, of which Google, Facebook, and LinkedIn are just a large sliver. Being capable and relevant in a world of technology generates a sizable portion of success.

"A well-designed day becomes the blueprint of your calendar for success."

— William B. Williams

The primary purpose of this book is to teach dentists to find success, to grow and improve their practices so that they have more free time and more profits. In that light, we often speak of the "$10,000-a-Day Dentist" because it is a convenient way to talk about service. Knowing our numbers, we can measure our success. Money is just a way to measure the level of service you provide. My wife Sheila says, "Serve people and the money will come." Putting it all into perspective, the Rotary International motto is "Service above Self."

The $10,000-a-Day Dentist

Design one day well, repeat it over and over, and soon you'll have a well-designed life. To create consecutive ten thousand-dollar days, a dentist must make declarations and decisions that reflect specific goals and values. The dentist must be dedicated and disciplined to do one day well so that a decade later, exceptional results occur. We only ever have today, one day, so make the most of each as it comes.

What does a $10,000-a-day dentist mean and where did that number come from? We'll discover that shortly. Right now, I want you to draw a line in the sand and declare these words: "I am a ten thousand dollar-a-day dentist. I break the chains that have bound me to the chair and kept me from achieving my fullest destiny. I place my signature at the end of this declaration, my personal declaration of independence."

Did you just read on or did you stop and make that declaration? Did you declare yourself a ten thousand dollar-a-day dentist? If not, do it now. The results five to ten years from now will bear testimony that you took the road less traveled but more beneficial. Writing a book on process for those whose mindsets are not on target is difficult. If I taught you sixteen chess moves without teaching you strategy, I would fail you as a mentor. You would never become a chess master. Likewise, as a dentist, I need to bring your mind up to speed before I can get your body into high gear.

It's time for a gift. I'm going to give you your official Swiss Army knife. Before you open it and begin to do amazing things, let's first read the instructions! This initial lesson is about your mental approach to highly productive dentistry. Follow me. Get ready for Truth Number One.

Truth Number One: Mindset

When you crack the code to become a big producer, you realize it's not that difficult. However, only a few ever produce in the five-figure range every day, week after week, month after month, year after year. Why is it such a struggle to be consistent? I believe it's because dentists don't plan well. They don't know what the BIG FIVE are, much less understand and achieve mastery over them.

Remember at the turn of the 20th century, when big game hunters used to go to Africa to bag the Big Five? They were after the fiercest, rarest, and most difficult kills on the continent: the rhino, the elephant, the lion, the leopard, and the Cape buffalo. Because we are now in a kinder, gentler time, we don't go to kill, only to enjoy. Now we go on safari in Kenya and Tanzania with telephoto lenses and digital cameras instead of rifles and bullets.

In dentistry, the Big Five are: (1) Mindset, (2) Team, (3) Facility, (4) Marketing, and (5) Capacity. To take down the Big Five, we need a hunter's mentality and strategic weapons. To own them and have command over them, we must become masters of our own selves. Stay tuned as we examine Mindset.

Mindset Matters Most

Don't let your mindset become a sunset, a daily disappearing act. Napoleon Hill said, "Whatever the mind of man can conceive and believe he can achieve." The mind of a successful businessman or woman must rise to the occasion daily. Dr. Ron McConnell, at Quest in 1981, taught me to picture my preferred reality. He opened my eyes to the world of possibility with the following story of a grasshopper.

With an audience of 567 dentists and dental team members at Quest 14, Ron began his lecture with a cartoon drawing of a bug in a jar, the lid screwed tightly shut. Ron contended that dental schools and dental societies train and govern their charges by limiting how high they can jump by keeping a lid on them. While enthusiastic grasshoppers will try to jump at first, they soon learn that it is painful to bump their heads on the lid, so they stop jumping as high. Conformity is the way to manage the masses, some say.

For a fortunate few, a giant comes along and removes the lid. Inspired by new teachings and insights into how the world can and does work the grasshopper leaps high once again, and in due time leaps from its jar, freed of all limitations. The story of the grasshopper was a watershed moment that set me free. That was the day I escaped dental school thinking and became a new type of dentist.

My next mentor, Dr. Omer K. Reed, offered a quote that I lived by for many years. It was, "If it's been done, it's probably possible." Omer authored the *International Newsletter*. I read it religiously for many years. In it, he brought forth ideas that shaped my career. He challenged my status quo and offered a better future to follow. And I did. If he had done it, I could, too. I took many of his Napili seminars and joined the Pentegra personal mastermind that he assembled in the 1980s. Those were the halcyon days of the first half of my dental career, before my halftime epiphany, my move to Suwanee, and my startup practice that I document in my book *Marketing the Million-Dollar Practice*.

The Mindset of Faith

Not every dentist chooses or gets to sit at the feet of a guru or mentor. Sometimes one has to go on faith because one has never seen or heard of a particular achievement. I had faith that if someone had done it, I could do the same thing. Romans 4:17 (RSV) reads, "God, who gives life to the dead and calls into existence the things that do not exist." It matters not that you've never done it before or that it hasn't ever been done. By having faith in your God-given ability, you can do it. So, if you declare that you are a ten thousand dollar-a-day dentist, it will come to pass if you implement steps that lead to your goal. Speak out and create the dynamics that begin as a seed and become reality in your life. It will happen.

Ten phrases encompass the mindset you'll need if you believe you can achieve your goal and declare the vision, mission, and culture:

1. Comprehensive dentistry
2. Team capability and delegation
3. Same-day dentistry – say yes
4. Patient focus – not self-focus
5. 100% Readiness – preparation
6. 100% Willingness – great attitude
7. Advance planning
8. Fees, financing, and family focus
9. 90-day goals
10. KPI and the Gold Key list

If you can wrap your head around these ten topics and understand them, you can become a ten thousand dollar-a-day dentist. The pages of this book will bring each of these topics into intense focus.

Truth Number Two: Facility

Bottlenecks are limitations in your ability to achieve your goals. Have you done an inventory of the bottlenecks in your life and practice? Your bottlenecks can be mental, physical, emotional, or spiritual. I'm going to focus on the physical bottlenecks that you can address to open the door to higher production. This is Truth Number Two.

To set the tone for success means your office has curb appeal, beautiful signage outside, and elegance in the reception area. Warm greetings come from the concierge. Our ten thousand dollar-a-day model revolves around the new patient experience – their tour of the office before our tour of their mouth, and the viewing of "what's on our walls" before being seated in the interview room to meet with the doctor. All these steps work in concert to create a powerful, positive impact on patients.

Because the future belongs to those prepared for change, a facility expansion plan should be in place to add multiple operatories as associate dentists are needed. The ideal ratio of operatories per dentist is five to one – three for the dentist and two for hygiene. As economy of scale becomes one of the major factors in success, dentists will begin to co-locate in groups more than ever before. This is the future of dentistry. That brings facility planning and construction into higher priority. The highly valued practice in the future will have seven to ten ops or more. Our current practice is fifteen ops, but it started out at five and grew to ten before settling into its current configuration. Furthermore, we have an expansion plan that can add up to five more operatories, including several surgical suites. Dental practices with great curb appeal and room to expand have a significant advantage over the competition. Plan to succeed when you plan your facility.

Technology is also a big part of the future with a stronger push for each practice to have a cone beam CT, dental lasers, CAD/CAM one-visit crowns, digital impressions, K-7 diagnostics, and T-Scan occlusal analysis. When doctors co-locate, they can jointly utilize those ultra-expensive gadgets and indispensable equipment. Reducing overhead by increasing group practice makes sense and saves cents.

Truth Number Three: Team

Teams come; teams go. Teams ebb and flow. What is consistent is change, and change is always a drain, an expense, and a trial. Building a highly productive, stable, and self-managed team will help you reach your goal. I call that "having a team of tens." Once you learn the truth about tens, you'll never want to practice any other way, and that is Truth Number Three.

Your team helps you to reach your goals and do what you do best – love and heal patients. To become a consistent ten thousand dollar-a-day dentist, you need a stable full of tens. They are self-managed, cross-trained partners who know how to convert patients from the hygiene room to restorative dentistry with the dentist. They know how to make a new patient exam appointment stretch to include big-ticket dentistry. And they do this because you, the dentist, delegate duties and have trained them to think independently and do their jobs well.

The ideal number of team members per dentist is six in most practices: two business assistants, two clinical assistants, and two hygienists. The more productive the dentist, the more likely they will employ additional business assistants and clinical assistants. As you go through this book, you will discover a multitude of ways you and your team can become more capable, more productive, and closer to the self-managed model we admire. Finally, you will discover ways to serve patients more efficiently. Once you learn and internalize these concepts and implement them, both dentist and dental team member will become tens. That's another reason we raise our glasses and say, "Great job, team!"

Truth Number Four: Marketing

Marketing well creates success. It's no secret. You need new patients in your practice to survive and thrive. What is the best way to attract them? What can you do to insure success in a highly competitive, dog-eat-dog world? Do you look at marketing as an expense or an investment? If your *return on investment*, or ROI, is negative, it's an expense. If it's positive, it's an investment. That's the truth you need to know about marketing. Only market what you know will give you a positive ROI.

Maintaining a healthy new patient influx is paramount to being consistently productive. Some practices average over a hundred new patients per dentist each month. Our practice averaged over a hundred new patients a month for the past fifteen years as we grew from one to four dentists. You need a fully integrated marketing action plan (MAP) that includes "the social six" (specific social media platforms) and local community "walkabout" by the dentist and the team to sustain new patient flow with a WebCentric focus.

As you read through these pages, you'll see that Alex the Guide defines each of the components of these five truths as he speaks with the five dentists and puts these truths into context.

Are You Influential?

A dentist must establish himself or herself as the expert and provide social proof that they can do what the patient wants with before and after photos, video interviews, and testimonials; and with written online reviews and print ads. Social proof and evidence of authority are major reputation enhancing needs for every practice and every doctor in the practice. Reputation management has become a major factor in practice success in this socially enlightened, Google-ized, Facebook world.

In my "Seven Mountains of Marketing" chapter in *Marketing the Million Dollar Practice*, I explain how a dental practice can become the leading influence in a community in each of seven distinct areas so that they dominate their competition. Those seven areas are education, government, economy, family, celebration, media, and religion. As dentists become involved in the community in each of these areas, their influence will double or triple. As influence grows, authority increases. As a result, referrals increase. You become the "go to" dentist in town. When you know about "Centers of Influence" and how to use them to your practice's advantage, you will recession-proof your practice.

Marketing the ten thousand dollar-a-day dentist becomes many times easier when the high-end niche patient funnel formula is used to draw in scores of patients who want dental implants, cosmetic makeovers, Invisalign, reconstructions, sedation dentistry, neuromuscular dentistry, and biologic dentistry. The funnel formula is a series of website landing pages, Facebook or Google ads, direct mail pieces, autoresponders, email series, videos, tracking software, and information delivery systems that are customized for each practice and dental service niche. Specifically, using predictive behavioral response techniques in directing our marketing message to ears that are ready to hear is what enables us to have a 75% better result than any other method of marketing. It is the wave of the future.

Marketing is one of the Big Five in dentistry, and too many dentists are not well-versed in understanding, setting-up, and running a strategic marketing plan. Dentists need to be involved in marketing their businesses if they want to succeed.

Truth Number Five: Capacity

Where does a dentist get the capacity to do better than average, more than other dentists commonly do? Deep down inside your heart, what's there? What are your core beliefs and how do you act upon them? Capacity is your ability to put it all together after all the training. I call it the heart of the matter and what separates the men from the boys and the women from the girls. Capacity in dentistry is that immeasurable quantity of toughness, grittiness, never-say-die determination to see it through to the end. Do you have the capacity or can you learn it and earn it? That is the Fifth Truth to discover.

Being a ten thousand dollar-a-day dentist is not for everyone. It is not easy. No one says dentistry has to be hard but it does take being a good multi-tasker to consistently hit the higher numbers. I believe it is far more likely you will become a high producer if you have many arrows in your quiver. The term "decathlon dentist" is appropriate: one who does all ten disciplines of dentistry (restorative, endo, ortho, TMD, implants, perio, fixed and removable prosthetics, oral surgery, and sedation). That means being able to provide multiple disciplines in one appointment for a single patient, using sedation as needed, and being efficient at work to the benefit of the patient, requiring fewer visits and less down time for the patient and the practice.

Systems make it all work, and well-documented patient care systems that run seamlessly and effortlessly will draw rave reviews and referrals from satisfied patients. A well-conceived treatment plan, executed painlessly in the time frame desired by the patient, often all in one day, will ultimately lead to you being consistently productive day after day. We simply do more in less time, while maintaining exceptional quality and service, and patients always appreciate that effort.

As we said at the outset, it's a mindset. If you have the team, the facility, the marketing, and the capacity to put it all together, you will be a consistent ten thousand dollar-a-day dentist. Following the Gold Key List (see Appendix 3), most any dentist can achieve that elusive goal.

If you want to soar like the eagle, perhaps the methods described in the following chapters are for you. I know from working with hundreds of dentists in internships, mentoring, associate-ships, and masterminds that not all are cut out to be a ten thousand dollar-a-day dentist. It takes a certain mindset, a concrete belief in oneself to go where most can't even imagine going. For those looking for a way to finish well, I offer another option to achieve that success. It's not an accident that you are reading this; it's providence. In time, you may have an amazing story to tell, and I invite you to share it with me.

Chapter 3

THE QUESTION

Alex was known as the Guide because he developed courses, wrote books, wrote chapters in books, wrote articles and manuals, produced videos, taught, lectured, and coached dentists all throughout his career. After six years in practice he began to lecture on TMD, head, neck, and facial pain and later orthodontics, orthopedics, occlusion, reconstruction, implants, and oral surgery. Later, after he had built a large practice, he began to teach on practice management and marketing, communication, leadership, and team building.

Over the years he had many students in his classes and workshops, his online classes and masterminds. The questions that always came up were "How do you do it? How are you so productive? How do you average such high production every day?" Alex looked over his last ten to fifteen years of practice and crunched the numbers. He had been keeping score, setting and recording goals each day, week, month, quarter, and year, so he knew what he had been doing. For the past twelve to thirteen years, he had averaged over ten thousand dollars a day in his operatories alone. He began to speak about how he repeatedly accomplished that goal. He taught other dentists how they, too, could average ten thousand dollars a day or more in their own practices. Alex presented a "Swiss Army knife" to those dentists who would listen.

The Socratic Method for Dentists

Alex credits Dr. Omer K. Reed with molding his mindset the most. He often advised, "If you must speak, ask questions." Omer was the modern day equivalent of Socrates, the Greek philosopher. Professor Rob Reich of the Stanford University Center for Teaching and Learning explained the Socratic method of teaching in Stanford University's newsletter on Teaching, Fall 2003, Vol. 13, No. 1- The Socratic Method: What it is and How to Use it in the Classroom:

In the Socratic method, the classroom experience is a shared dialogue between teacher and students in which both are responsible for pushing the dialogue forward through questioning. The "teacher," or leader of the dialogue, asks probing questions in an effort to expose the values and beliefs which frame and support the thoughts and statements of the participants in the inquiry. The students ask questions as well, both of the teacher and each other.

Alex the guide learned to ask questions and dig deeper when asked a question. He focused on setting the stage and letting the student wander about, exploring and discovering the acres of "diamonds" buried in the fields beneath their feet. Alex knew that while there was nothing new on the earth, many merely trod, laboriously plowing the field above the gems at their disposal. They never stopped to look for the one thing that would lead them to a breakthrough.

To those who asked, "How do you produce ten thousand dollars a day?" Alex answered, "Depends on where you are in your career."

What makes sense to a mature dentist will not apply equally to a young dentist. Experience matters. It influences perspective. Generally speaking, Alex broke down the Five Truths and applied them to each of the five periods of a dentist's life. Every dentist must eventually assimilate strength in all five truth categories to have a highly successful and productive practice.

"Patience, persistence, and perspiration make an unbeatable combination for success," said Napoleon Hill. Indeed, the combination is a formidable obstacle for young dentists to overcome. Many want it all now. Alex preached patience as well as persistence. He knew that what was worth attaining was worth never giving up on, never quitting because the work became too difficult. Painstaking persistence leads to success. Alex knew what each of these five dentists needed, and when the timing was right, he would share the missing key with them. Many times, the way a person discovers a hidden truth dictates the value they place upon it.

The Missing Key

For the young dentist, such as Dr. Blair Bennett, mindset was the truth she needed to understand. Preparing the mind involves two paradigm shifts. The first shift opens the mind to new ideas that may seem incongruent to one's upbringing at home or in the classroom. Gather all of the necessary components (beliefs, attitudes, and concepts) for success in the beginning so that you get the desired outcome. Mindset is where one can get it completely wrong or completely right and starting out on the wrong foot leads to futility. Asking the right questions early in one's career is wise.

For the local dentist, such as Dr. Jack Mudd, who had been in practice for many years, the Team Truth was the most important. Eventually, all successful dentists must rely on their teams to achieve success. Investing in workplace collaborators who share the same vision, mission, and culture will pay significant dividends to those who understand the power of teamwork. Jack found that relying on others could bring freedom. Doing everything yourself and not delegating duties leads to stasis and places limitations on growth. Alex gave Dr. Mudd a can opener from his Swiss Army knife, so that he could open up and become more available to his team and his patients.

A servant dentist like Dr. Edward Boyle, who had ten years in practice, gained the most from the Facility Truth. Most dentists don't think about their facilities in the long term, decades out from their beginnings. Yet this could largely determine how well a dentist finishes. The facility often limits one's ability to expand and grow, even when there is a desire to do so. Dr. Boyle wanted to travel and experience more than life at the dental chair. Planning for facility expansion and a team of doctors in advance expedites the transition from solo to group practice. Increased efficiency could provide Dr. Boyle the opportunity to reach his goals.

A peak performance dentist like Dr. Carley Matthews would benefit from knowing and applying Marketing Truth to her already excellent practice. When one has all the clinical tools in hand to do a superb job yet lacks the raw materials needed to assemble and create one's masterpiece, growth is stunted. A factory needs a good supply chain to feed its production. Likewise, a dental practice needs a well-oiled marketing machine to feed it. There is nothing sadder than a highly skilled dentist sitting idle, playing Solitaire on their iPhone waiting on patients to call for an appointment. Alex believed in being proactive and encouraged creating an effective marketing action plan as the answer to her biggest need.

Dr. Steve Blake, the mature dentist, would reach his potential by applying Capacity Truth to his practice. Margaret Atwood, in *Cat's Eye* says, "Potential has a shelf life." Zig Ziglar links the word potential with passion, saying, "When you catch a glimpse of your potential, that's when passion is born." Passion expressed in dentistry leads to higher capacity. Steve began to realize his dreams when he understood the way a dentist achieves capacity. A lifetime of training points to a time when the dentist is fully engaged to create their masterpiece, their pièce de résistance.

The Austrian Thing

Alex, to give more specific advice and counsel, would often sit with a dentist at local Starbucks coffee shops and do "the Austrian thing." The Kaffeehauses of Vienna are a centuries-old tradition, a monument to the fruitful wasting of time on the one hand and a hangout for building deeper relationships on the other. The fluid character of the social space was the perfect place to find and explore intellectual and creative stimulation. What better place to ask questions? Time stands still, the world grows strangely dim, and the mind takes flight, able to explore mysteries, purposes, and motivations. Sometimes a dentist needs to get away from the familiar sounds and smells of the dental office and do "the Austrian thing."

What questions arose when Alex met with each doctor? What questions have begun to arise in your mind? What dreams have begun to stir in your heart? Wouldn't you like to get your hands on your own dental Swiss Army knife?

Chapter 4

THE SERVANT DENTIST, DR. EDWARD BOYLE

Alex sat with Dr. Edward Boyle in the Java House, in Nairobi, Kenya. They had landed at Kenyatta airport the night before, stayed overnight at the Methodist Guest House in the posh Lavington district, and were awaiting the arrival of other mission team members from the US on British Air. They began to talk dentistry, and pretty soon the question came up. "How do you do what you do so consistently?"

Alex answered by asking Dr. Boyle, "Why do you want to know? Why is it important to you to be more productive? What is success to you?"

As they talked, the focus began to revolve around having time to do the things Edward wanted to do. His interests were many; his passion was great for serving others, and being mission-minded topped the list.

Alex asked, "Ed, how much free time is enough?"

If you want a fulfilled life, you need a schedule that allows you to be fulfilled in each area of your life. If you need more time for your passion, then you need to find a way to support your "free time activities" with your "productive time activities." Edward needed to solve the engineering issues of being productive as a dentist so that he could also be productive in the social and spiritual arena. With this in mind, Alex began to develop a prescription for success for Dr. Boyle.

THE TOUR – THE NPE

"What can I do to get to the next level?" Edward asked.

Alex knew that to be successful, dentists and team members have to connect with patients on the first visit. It sets the stage for all else. Borrowing from Shakespeare, Alex explained that if life is but a play and we are all actors, then one of the most important scenes is your New Patient Experience (NPE). We look at the NPE as a scene with a script, with actors coming on stage at the proper times, on cue at the right moment. The result of the NPE and the New Patient Tours of the office is definitive.

The tour of your office with your new patient coordinator establishes that you are unique. Your expertise is showcased by demonstrated social proof on the walls. The goal of the tour is to develop a rapport and to listen to and understand what drives and motivates a patient.

The NPE has five parts: (1) the greeting; (2) the tour; (3) the interview; (4) the examination, and (5) the release. Just like in big game fishing, you want the new patient to be released from the practice unharmed, willing to return. Your intent should be to deliver a Tony Award-winning performance with your team each day for every new patient, establishing bonds of trust and rapport.

With Alex's description of the New Patient Experience, Edward saw that he could grow his practice to the next level by engaging his patients in a more personal and in-depth manner. Alex was right that this would make it easier to treat patients when their wishes were more completely understood. Dr. Boyle appreciated fully the "It's not about me; it's about them."

SEVEN MOUNTAINS OF MARKETING

Edward's next question was "What's the next thing to focus on at this stage of my career?"

Alex said that influential people were twice as successful as those who had no sway. He outlined a system for gaining momentum for practice growth that would become unstoppable – the Seven Mountain Strategy. It's all about influence. If you want to be successful, you need to be in a position to influence your community in positive ways. One way is for them to recognize you and your practice as one of the top dental practices in the region. Alex explained his theory about centers of influence and how they come into play with a dental practice's marketing efforts.

Alex had read *The Seven Mountain Prophesy*, by Johnny Enlow, that led him to develop the Seven Mountains marketing strategy. The strategy illustrates that Edward needs to be perceived as the most influential dentist in seven specific areas:

1. Government
2. Education
3. Media
4. Economy or business
5. Family
6. Celebration or entertainment
7. Religion

When you are the "go to" guy or gal in one or more of these areas of influence, you influence the actions and thoughts of a segment of society. Becoming a leader in any one area allows you to influence that group when it comes to dentistry.

People naturally flock to and defer to leaders. Your stock rises, and in time, so will your practice.

Alex recommended Edward study Chapter 33 of *Marketing the Million Dollar Practice* and the Seven Mountains of marketing and become more influential in his community.

EFFICIENCY SYSTEMS & KPI

Obviously, doing what Alex suggested would make Edward more effective and bring in more patients through referrals. Being busier was a good thing, but it created a crunch when there were too many patients demanding appointments.

"When do you know it's time to add an associate?" asked Edward. "I'm working as quickly and efficiently as I can, and we still have patients who can't get an appointment for several weeks because we are so booked."

Alex had worked with over eighteen associates and had been one himself, so he had great insights. It is time to add an associate when you have maximized your capacity to produce. Are you as effective and efficient as you can be? Is there more that could be done if there were more hands on deck? Take a step back and look at what other dentists do. Sometimes only a mental bottleneck keeps you stuck at a particular level in your practice.

Why is one dentist twice as fast as another dentist? Why aren't all dental teams capable of operating at the same speed? The answers lie in mindset and expectations. If you believe it's possible, you'll be able to do it. If you've heard it or seen it done, you may be able to do it. Some dentists need to be given permission to do more than they think possible. They need to establish a new mental paradigm.

One of the best "A-ha!" moments a dentist can have is when he or she sees another dentist do crown preps in ninety seconds, a root canal in twenty minutes, or a full-mouth reconstruction of twenty-eight crowns in four or five hours without losing focus on excellence. Aristotle said, "Excellence is never an accident. It is always the result of high intention, sincere effort, and intelligent execution; it represents the wise choice of many alternatives. Choice, not chance, determines your destiny." If it's been done, it's probably possible. Make your systems efficient and you will do more in less time.

Once the dentist believes this truth, he or she must pass it on to the team. Expectations must be established before they can be met. Efficient methods must be developed, documented, and adhered to by the team. What gets measured gets done, so it is critical to measure your key performance indicators, your KPI. Getting to the top takes time and effort, but once at the top, staying there is not so challenging. Develop efficient dental systems and measure the KPI. Once you know your numbers, you can compare them to what has been done by others. And as Zig Ziglar says, "I'll see you at the top!"

Alex addressed the question of adding an associate next. There are two reasons to hire an associate. The first is to take stress from the owner and distribute the workload. The second is to increase profits. When you have maximized your efficiency and can't do more, it may be time to look for an additional set of hands. One reason to get an associate is to create more free time. Carve a place for the associate out of your patient base or increase marketing to build a new patient base. Alex always added dentists ahead of the need and marketed them into success. Edward determined that he was ready for an associate.

100% READINESS

Dr. Edward Boyle said, "My team stresses me out more than my patients. How do I overcome that?"

Edward was the tail of the dog, getting wagged by the team, at the mercy of what they did or did not do. His prescription for success was to tighten some screws that had loosened with his Swiss Army knife. He discussed his outlook on expectations of his own practice. "When I go into work every morning, I plan to maximize my time and eliminate wasted moments. I want to be productive from the start of my day until the end. I've been called a machine, but that's just how I'm wired. I want to get it done the best, most efficient way I can! One way to achieve maximum efficiency and keep the flow smooth is for everyone on my team to be 100% ready for the procedure I am to perform. Rooms, tray setups, equipment, computers, and even the patients have to be ready for me to begin my work. Finances and insurance questions must be handled and which teeth or procedure we plan to do that day must be clear before the doctor enters the room. I like it when the papers (informed consents, financial agreements, and post-operative instructions) are signed, the anesthetic syringe is loaded, and my patient is reclined in the chair, ready to go.

"One of the tenets in our practice is that everything should be done to remove obstacles that interfere with the doctor doing his or her duty, which is to love and heal patients. Being 100% ready to go is a mindset that enables this to happen multiple times every day."

Alex averages twenty to thirty patients in a typical busy day, including checking hygiene patients. How would you like to have twenty perfect beginnings a day? How would you feel if you had twenty slightly off-target starts? Wouldn't that feel like a disruption? The team that prepares and is 100% ready is the team Alex wants. How about you?

Chapter 5

THE
PEAK PERFORMANCE DENTIST, DR. CARLEY MATTHEWS

Before there was Starbucks, there was Metro Coffee House on Broad Street, in Augusta. The first AAID Maxi-Course was in progress at the Medical College of Georgia, and attendees often started their days by gathering at the landmark coffee shop for lively discussion. Dr. Carley Matthews, from Marietta, Georgia, was enrolled in the course, as was Alex. They sat in a quiet corner and talked implants, bone grafting, and the like before the conversation got around to her practice. She asked Alex how she could be more like him.

She was an accomplished clinician who could go far in her career. He understood some of her goals and what seemed to drive her. His question to her was simple. "What are your career goals?" With peak-performer dentists the question is always where are they headed and how and when will they know they have reached that place.

Alex had seen many dentists go through the Roman candle experience: on fire with a big bang early in their career, only to flame out in a sputtering whimper after a short while. Their focus was not placed correctly to develop strong family bonds; cultivate a circle of friends, guides, and accountability partners; or nurture an intimate relationship with their spiritual father. The singular focus on becoming top guns had led many promising dentists to wasting chunks of their lives because they had to start over multiple times.

Alex then asked, "How do you spell balance in your life?" Alex shared a personal experience demonstrating that those who burned the candle at both ends sometimes exploded too soon. Finding balance is an important step in finding success.

Dr. Matthews shared where she wanted to go in dentistry and why she was driven to reach the highest echelons of the profession. She had a level head and would make it, thought Alex. Ready to get on with the first step, Alex gave Carley a thumbs-up.

ADVANCE PLANNING

"What challenges will I face over the next ten years and how do I avoid problems?" Carley asked Alex.

"Most dentists do not design their futures," explained Alex. "Most just show up to work and let it happen. William Jennings Bryant said, 'Destiny is not a matter of chance; it is a matter of choice. It is not a thing to be waited for; it is a thing to be achieved.' Most dentists don't spend enough time envisioning, goal-setting, and preparing for the future; they spend most of their time busy in the present. One way to break that habit is to schedule time to work on their business, not just in their business."

Alex presented Carley with this prescription for success: "Plan your year. Plan your quarter. Plan your month. Plan your week. Plan your day. And plan each patient's appointments. Each segment of time must be planned to achieve the $10,000-a-day average.

"Setting goals and having a strategic plan sets up the big picture, the macro version of your practice success plan. But as your time grows shorter, it becomes even more critical to develop the micro aspects of your plan. As they say, 'God is in the details.' You have to make everything come together with Swiss precision. Attention paid to small things yields big rewards. If you plan each day, the big plan will take care of itself. What you do every day creates your win as much as the strategic plan you generate yearly. That's why," Alex continued, "I focus on achieving one excellent day at a time. Just give all your energy to making the perfect day. Omer Reed taught us to value the $5000 day because the $5000-day dentist would become a million-dollar producer by working a full two hundred days a year. Once you know how to do that you can repeat it over and over again. This is how the concept of the $10,000-a-day dentist came into existence. I thought to myself, 'I've done this for the past twelve years. What do I do to accomplish a great day every day? How can I share it with other dentists so that they can do the same thing?' All the pieces need to be on the table to play the game. It's eight AM. Do you have all the pieces and are you ready to play?"

MASTERMINDS MAXIMIZE CAPACITY

Carley liked that exchange because it showed her how to create the result she had always dreamed of. "How do I go from a two million-dollar practice to a four million-dollar practice?" she asked.

Not many dentists think like that, but those who do can do it. The size of your practice is only limited by the mind. Dentistry is a series of interactions. The student learns from his professors and applies what he learned on his patients. A dentist learns from her advanced general practice residency and applies what she learned on her patients. An experienced dentist moves up the ladder of success in CE (continuing education) courses, one symposium at a time, adding to his repertoire. The king of dental learning experiences is the dental mastermind. In the mastermind, an experienced mentor brings to the table like-minded dentists who want to grow their practices by sharing what they have learned over a lifetime of CE and patient treatment episodes.

Alex said, "Masterminds have given my practice its biggest boosts. That's why I've been a part of seven or eight masterminds over my forty-year career. Now, I delight in being "the guide," putting together and leading dental masterminds, so that others can achieve the same results I have achieved in my career. Doctors who participate in masterminds often double their practices, so it's conceivable that a two million-dollar practice could grow into a four million-dollar practice over a three-to-five-year period. One thing about a mastermind is that the dentists all support one another. They cheer each other on, announcing best days and best months with pride and joy, and know that others will celebrate with them, not begrudge their success. I like to say 'they trumpet their success as they trump their local competitors.'"

FEES, FINANCING AND FAMILY FOCUS

Most dentists would not think Dr. Matthews had any problems or issues left to overcome. But as a forward-thinking entrepreneur, she asked more questions. "What are some of the pitfalls to avoid as I climb the ladder of success?"

Alex replied, "I come from an abundance mentality, not a scarcity mentality. So as we develop our $10,000-a-day abundance model, we need to focus on fees and financing in our practices. It would be wise to unchain our minds from the belief that all decisions made by patients are based on cost. Value is equally important to most patients, especially those seeking high-end dentistry.

"Two points are worth noting," Alex continued. "Marketing creates value and establishes you as the expert and the authority in your area for fine dentistry. Let that mindset be yours when you market so that it will also be the patients' when they arrive at your practice. This same mindset will be particularly beneficial when they are listening to the treatment proposal. Your marketing look and feel establishes who you are to the public. If you want to attract high-end patients, you have to model successful, high-end businesses. Curb appeal, elegant interior décor, and professional appearance matters.

"Behind closed doors, in the room with your patient treatment coordinator during case presentation, even a well-heeled person will appreciate the ability to finance dental work. Always have a financing option for your patients. I'm not talking about in-house financing. I do not advocate being a bank for your patients. They need to utilize third-party financing options, like Care Credit or The Lending Tree. Creative financing will provide the profits you need to pay handsome bonuses to your team and provide a fat retirement fund for you and your family.

"Don't be a stranger. The more you bring people into your inner circle at the new patient experience and let them know who you are as you speak with them and find out who they are, the more they will consider you 'family.' When they see you as family, they may loosen their focus on money and let value be the deciding factor. People ask how much a crown is when they don't know you or know what else to say. Once they are comfortable with you and the practice, they say, 'Doc, what would you do if you were me?' This is when they feel like family and trust you implicitly. Our goal is to attract discriminating individuals who want and can afford fine dentistry and who become like family once they have joined us."

PATIENT TREATMENT COORDINATOR

Carley asked, "What makes dentistry at this high level easy?"

Alex considered one of the keys to his success. For over thirty years, he had not done consults with his patients. "Every team needs a closer," he said. "The patient treatment coordinator is our closer and a very effective one. Of course, we need an able-bodied, cross-trained backup, but this staffer does most treatment plan presentations. This is true for all doctors in the practice, from the most grizzled veteran to the brand-new baby docs. The ace case presentation specialist does all the selling. When this patient treatment coordinator system is combined with the new patient experience system, the acceptance rate of the treatment is nearly the same for all doctors – very high. Typically, the doctor is designated as the closer, especially in young practices, but is he or she the best for the job?

"I would argue that there is a better person to do it for two main reasons. The doctor's time is better spent doing what only he or she can legally do – diagnosing, drilling, cutting, extracting, or implanting. Do you know how many crown preps a typical dentist can do in one hour? The team's job is to keep the dentist busy doing what makes the most sense...and cents.

"When the sole job of a team member is to sell and close cases, staying focused for as long as it takes to gain rapport, listen well, understand, show empathy, and explain all treatment options and the various insurance and financing ramifications, the doctor is freed to do his or her job. Also, when there is no perceived personal gain, a patient in the consultation room will feel that the patient treatment coordinator has their best interests at heart. And it's true. They do."

Chapter 6

THE YOUNG DENTIST, DR. BLAIR BENNETT

The 1818 Club sits atop the Gwinnett Chamber of Commerce building on Sugarloaf Drive in Duluth, GA. It's not a public place like a Starbucks, but the coffee is excellent and the ambience is perfect for interviewing prospective dental associates. Members of the 1818 business club are focused on greasing the wheels of commerce. It's good to be a part of the inner circle.

Alex is an 1818 member and suggested the club as a meeting spot. Dr. Blair Bennett had met Alex at the Atlanta Craniomandibular Society meeting a few months back and hoped to become an associate in Alex's practice. Alex had conversed with Dr. Konzelman, Blair's dental school professor, and he knew that Blair was interested in the neuromuscular concept of occlusion and what he had been doing in his practice for many years.

Some dental graduates come out of school looking for a place to work. Any employment will do. Others have thought about the path they wish to climb. Blair knew she wanted to focus on the whole person, not just teeth. She already understood, from her studies in oral medicine and diagnosis that body health is connected to oral health.

Sometimes being laser-focused on a goal at an early age can be like wearing blinders that hinder one's growth and development, so Alex asked, "What are your hopes and dreams, Blair?" He wanted to know what mattered in her life beyond dentistry. A career must be built on passion and it must come from deep within, so that the fire does not ebb for lack of fuel. Dr. Bennett contemplated and answered the question as best she could, and Alex asked another question, one that often stymies young dentists. "What would you do if you had enough money? If you were capable of doing what you really want to do, what would it be? If you were free to do anything you want, what would it be?"

Blair gave the question serious thought. Putting goals down on paper, making lists, and coming back to review those lists every week, is a skill that many young dentists never acquire. Going a step further, Alex suggested she create a vision board. Find her dream house, dream vacation, dream practice facility, dream spouse, and dream income level in photograph form and then cut them out or make drawings and mount them on a poster board. A vision board is a mental activation tool that creates movement in one's life.

COMPREHENSIVE DENTISTRY

Dr. Bennett asked, "What is your best piece of advice for me as a new dentist?"

"Successful dentists have a particular mindset, one that says, 'I am capable and I am confident,'" said Alex. "They also believe in comprehensive dentistry for their patients. They diagnose everything they see no matter what the patient's status or current interest appears to be. The comprehensive dentist examines thoroughly, diagnoses completely, and prescribes treatment plans that are comprehensive. Education matters because you can't diagnose what you don't know, what you don't see, or what you don't understand. Plus, in too many cases, a dentist will only develop a treatment plan for what they can do, paying little attention to TMD, perio, ortho, or the need for implants because they don't know how to provide that service or don't want to refer the patient out for that treatment. It puts a great deal of pressure on the dentist. Dental schools only prepare us to do the basics, so it is important to be a life-long learner. As you learn, you will become a master dentist. Your treatment plans will become more complex.

"So what is the big take-away? Education and experience matter. Decide that all patients deserve the best and will receive comprehensive dentistry. Comprehensive dentistry is always best for the patient. When I meet with new patients, I tell them that I will give them a thorough examination, and from that I will develop for them a five-year plan. I give them permission to complete the plan in as little as one visit, if it is possible, or in ten years, depending on what they prefer and can afford. There should be no surprises when the entire case is planned and presented upfront.

Blair got the message; education must be a life-long activity. One is not done when the diploma is handed over at the end of four years of dental school. Blair had not realized that the complexity of the cases she could handle would largely determine her entire career.

SAME DAY DENTISTRY – SAY YES

Blair frowned contemplatively. "What's the first thing you'd do if you were me, given the stage of my career?" "Easy question to answer," thought Alex. The need to get busy fast was imminent.

Alex began to describe a system. "Young dentists don't generally have a book of patients on which to work," said Alex. "They have no history in practice. They are an unknown. That means they don't get many referrals from satisfied patients. There is no backlog of people waiting to come in. What are they to do? All new dentists must work on strangers. They have to be creative and able to handle dental emergencies. They have to be able to convert a dental shopper into a satisfied patient. They have to learn to 'Wow' them on the spot or risk losing them to the practice down the street. Conversion becomes a vital skill to learn.

"One of my biggest mindset shifts of the last decade was focusing on saying 'yes' to same day dentistry. Whatever I can do today, I will. When there is a willing patient and we can create time in the schedule, we say yes. When I'm in the hygiene room checking a patient, I might say, 'If we can work it into our schedule, Mrs. Jones, would you like to get that done today,' if I know my schedule and I have a team capable of spontaneous changes.

"Throughout the day, we try to fill in the holes that show up in our schedules in the doctor's operatories and hygiene. We work to engineer the best production possible and exceed our daily goals. It's a mindset of abundance and opportunity, rather than scarcity and limitations. Being patient-focused and saying yes results in increased production and return business, as well as increased referrals because your team is flexible (mindset), cross-trained, and has a can-do attitude toward meeting the patients' needs. Everything is connected. There are no insular events in a well-run practice. Once the gestalt of the new patient's experience is understood, the pace of advancement accelerates. Gestalt is a set of things such as a person's thoughts and experiences considered as a whole and regarded as amounting to more than the sum of its parts. When the entire crew of the dental practice has bought into the vision, mission, and culture of the practice and utilizes the tools and techniques of good communication, the experience that the patients receive goes beyond what is normal in dentistry. This perception of excellence creates the wow factor.

"For experienced dentists with a fairly solid book of patients, this opens the door to higher productivity by allowing the team to fill in any holes in the schedule. For young dentists with no patients, this is the means to survival. They must make hay with the opportunities before them: re-care patients, emergency patients, and new patients. Excellence in communication, listening, and gaining instant rapport are skills all new dentists must learn. Have you looked carefully at the barriers to delivering dental care? Eliminate them and see your productivity flourish."

MARKETING ACTION PLAN (MAP)

Dr. Blair Bennett, our "baby doc," knew she would have to do a lot of work to sell herself to people with whom she had no history. That is the nature of being a new associate in a practice. Thinking of the next step she asked, "Where do I need to focus my attention in order to have a strong, highly productive practice?"

"Christopher Columbus didn't have a map, so he didn't end up where he thought he was going. If you want to go to East India instead of the Americas, you need a plan. In marketing, we call that a MAP, a *marketing action plan.* To be a $10,000-a-day dentist, you will need fifty to a hundred new patients a month in the beginning and twenty to forty new patients a month to maintain that level of production once your practice is mature.

"The marketing action plan spells out what you'll do to attract those new patients. Marketing is not an expense. It is an investment. The more you invest, the greater your rate of growth. Keeping track of the return of investment is important so that you can double up on the winning strategies and cut the losers. A good marketing action plan has nine steps and should be able to be written in nine sentences. It should be one page in length, simple and understandable. The purpose of the marketing action plan is to clarify who you are. This keeps the focus on what is important and helps you and your team stay on message. Consider this a blueprint of a MAP by filling in the blanks."

Alex scribbled a few sentences on a sheet of paper and handed it to Blair.

1. The specific purpose of my marketing is to ________ .
2. The competitive advantage we want to stress is ______.
3. Our unique selling proposition is __________.
4. Our target audience is __________ .
5. The marketing weapons we will use are __________.
6. Our market niche is __________.
7. Our identity is __________.
8. Our marketing budget is ____________ percentage of our production.
9. Our implementation plan is to ______________.

"If you get each step right, there will be plenty of patients knocking on your door. To set up your marketing action plan, work with experienced marketers who have done successful dental marketing. When I started my practice," Alex reflected, "I read *Guerrilla Marketing*, by J. Conrad Levinson. Later, I read *Marketing the Million-Dollar Practice: 28 Ways to Grow Your Practice One-Half Million Dollars a Year.* From the insights I gained, I built my practice to over five million dollars in production in just a few years. If you have a MAP, you can reach the goals you set."

IDEAL NUMBER OF TEAM MEMBERS PER DENTIST

Blair imagined a time when enough new patients was not the issue. "What pitfalls do I need to avoid once marketing kicks in and new patient flow is high? What could hinder my progress?"

"How many team members does it take to support a $10,000-per-day dentist? That sounds like the lead-in to a joke, but the punch line is no joke. It takes the number you need. Not all dentists are created equally. Each rises to his own level of clinical awareness, clinical excellence, leadership ability, managerial acuity, and drive to succeed.

"Once I was a judge in the Small Business Person of the Year competition at our local Chamber of Commerce, having been the winner the previous year," said Alex. "One candidate, another dental company, was up for the award. Their statistics were submitted and one number stood out to me: revenue vs. number of employees. They produced $100,000 per employee per year. Our practice the year prior had produced $200,000 per employee per year. In dentistry, standards show that the average practice production is $100,000 per employee, with a good number being $150,000 per employee.

"Take a snapshot of your practice. If you are on the lower side of this reference number, are you overstaffed, or are you under-producing as a team? If you are on the upper side of this equation, you are setting a new standard for excellence. If you are setting record numbers, has your team been sharing in the rewards? The obvious truth is that a $10,000-a-day dentist is going to have a well-compensated team. The pitfall for many dentists is being improperly staffed," said Alex. "Either there are too many staff members for the production or too few staff, creating a bottleneck that hinders production."

Chapter 7

THE MATURE DENTIST, DR. STEVE BLAKE

When dentists get near the end of their careers, a fatalistic point of view begins to creep into their thinking. They start looking at playing their last hand. Dr. Steve Blake was like that, except he was not yet ready to hang it up. He did not have enough saved for retirement to give him the choices for which he had hoped. Some of that came from living a lifestyle of affluence but not investing like the affluent. Fortunately, old dogs can learn new tricks…lots of them.

During their first session, Alex asked, "Steve, how much is enough?"

Unless one knows what is needed to retire with a certain income, one is never capable of retiring. As a dentist works towards the decision to slow down or retire, he needs to know his goal for savings and what the yearly income from his investments will be.

Steve shared his numbers, and Alex asked, "How does producing more help you achieve your goal?" Alex knew that stating a goal would not make it happen, but it was the first step. Once the goal was known, the work needed to take place. For Steve, all that was needed was a heavy dose of mindset updating and the Capability Truth. Experienced dentists with good practices can magnify their results effortlessly and predictably with a change in mindset and a few key tactics that unlock the hidden treasure in their practices. Once dentists like Steve see a Swiss Army knife, they intuitively know what to do with it.

GOALS AND RESULTS

Alex works with many dentists in the golden years of their practices and he has seen many of them do well with his guidance. Conversely, he has seen a few who do not heed or value his advice. They continue to muddle along, sliding miserably into their retirement. Alex has a prescription for those who want to finish well, as Dr. Steve Blake did.

"What do I do if I'm old enough to retire but can't or don't want to quite yet?" asked Steve. A goal well stated was a goal half-solved, so Alex moved in that direction, helping Steve to clarify what he wanted.

"A goal worth setting is a goal worth reaching," said Alex. "Grab the bull by the horns, and most times you'll exceed your goals. That's the reason to focus on your daily goal and your eight AM goal. Most people have figured out that a daily goal, such as ten thousand dollars, is a good thing, but how many have an eight o'clock goal, too? I call it right at eight. When I drive by the office on my days off, I want to see eight patients' cars in the parking lot at eight o'clock – two for each dentist and one for each hygienist. When I'm working, I want to achieve my personal eight AM goal, which is three in three every day. That means three patients in three operatories at eight AM. My team knows my goals and focuses on them to start every day on an ideal note. Remember, we can only do what we can do right now.

Tomorrow will never come, and yesterday is lost. Benjamin Franklin said, 'Never put off until tomorrow what you can do today.'

"Your goal may be a one, two, three, or five million-dollar practice, but to get there you must divide the whole year into parts. We build the numbers one day at a time. In our practice, every person has goals, not just the dentist. When everyone consistently hits their daily goals, we exceed our big goal. We get the result we want. The big take-away today is this," said Alex. "With goals, start from the end and work backward, accomplish your micro goals every day, and you will win big in the end. By maximizing each day, you'll finish well at year's end."

SYSTEMS

Steve had not heard of having an eight AM goal in addition to a daily goal, so he was excited to implement that in his practice. It could be done on Monday and would take no real planning. He just had to state his goal and make it happen with a lot of effort and desire.

"What if I need to grow my retirement account? How can I maximize my practice?" asked Steve.

"It's never too late to create and start running systems. The answer to your question involves creating patient care systems. Systems create wealth. Ask Henry Ford about his production system. Ask Bill Gates about his operating system. Ask Julia Child about her recipe system. Ask Richard Branson about his entrepreneurial system. All will say that their secret to wealth was creating and following a system. Patient care systems are a significant part of the $10,000-a-day dentist's strategic plan. They carefully outline the steps for every procedure performed in the practice. There is no creating it on the fly, no winging it, and no last minute planning in a well-oiled practice."

Examples of a patient care system would include:

1. The dental emergency appointment
2. The new patient experience
3. The VIP consult (which is a free second opinion consultation)
4. CMO exam – the craniomandibular orthopedic workup
5. 21-Point smile analysis – the cosmetic evaluation
6. Periodontal – oral – systemic connection treatment protocol
7. Dental implant exam and diagnosis appointment with the cone beam CT scan
8. Full-mouth reconstruction pre-planning appointment
9. Full-mouth reconstruction appointment
10. Invisalign exam and impression appointment

"Every procedure is a system and every appointment follows a system," said Alex. "Imagine having a system to diagnose a problem and plan a solution. Then imagine your business assistants using a system to get the patient into that treatment and the clinical assistants implementing a system to do that work without additional input from you, the dentist. Now imagine that for every procedure, every patient, every day. Would stress in the office be lower, production higher, and profits magnified? The answer is always yes. Having patient care systems in place all across the practice is like everyone on the team having their own Swiss Army knife, ready to handle anything, anytime, anywhere."

PREPLANNING

Steve was getting excited. He saw the impact of what he was being shown. It really wasn't new. It was mostly replacing an outdated mindset with something that had been done successfully by a handful of highly productive dentists. Steve was ready to grab the bull by the horns and make it work. "What should I focus on in order to finish well?" he asked.

"How can one dentist do $10,000 every day in his or her operatory? We do it by having a master plan laid out a year in advance, a strong ninety-day plan for the quarter, and a daily plan that includes ways to make up for any difference in the actual scheduled dentistry versus the $10,000 goal."

Benjamin Franklin has been credited with saying, 'To fail to plan is to plan to fail.'

"In my practice, every day starts with a fully-attended, to-the-point, structured morning huddle where we launch our $10,000 day. A pod is a doctor and his or her dental auxiliary. In a small practice, everyone attends the same meeting. As multiple doctors enter the practice, the pods split into doctor-led groups for the morning huddle. Each team member in a pod reports vital information about the patients they will see, including medical history, family news, current appointment specifics, and what kind of future treatment are still pending. The business assistant tells us about each new patient, relating information they gathered on the initial phone call about their visit. They announce yesterday's production and collection numbers, today's numbers, and any opportunities to fill in or enhance our day. The clinical assistants tell us about pending treatment and today's work because we are concerned with bringing the patient to a successful completion of their dentistry. We want to be prepared for the 'What's next?' discussion at the end of their appointment. The doctor and the clinical assistant plan for the next appointment as they complete the current appointment, verbalizing the benefit of getting it done and the length of time it will take. They resell the case at each appointment and continually overcome objections. Patients are always looking to delay treatment, and that is never in their best interest. We have to remain their therapeutic advocate.

"Dental hygienists tell us about their patients and all of their diagnosed and planned dental work. Because we believe in same day dentistry and 'just say yes,' the hygienists aim to fill any open spot in our schedule with one of their patients. Likewise, we look to fill any open hygiene spots from our doctors' patient schedule. And the key," said Alex, "is this: we dissect the day. We plan for success because we have all pre-planned our days."

DELEGATION AND COMMUNICATION

Dr. Steve Blake knew that creating a busier and more productive schedule would risk overworking and stressing out. "How can I be highly productive yet have balance, too?" Steve asked.

Alex had already worked through this problem himself. "You've heard the old saying," he said. "'Many hands make light work.' That is the secret of delegation. Move duties to those who can do it faster, cheaper, or more effectively. By reducing the load on the most highly paid member of the team – you – you can take on more pressing duties and ultimately be more productive.

"Getting the doctor to the next place he or she needs to be, on time, should be the team's priority. Getting the doctor there with all the knowledge about what the patient needs and expects would be an added bonus. That's why it's necessary to make use of a communication tool for doctors as they travel between rooms. I use route cards. When route cards are used efficiently, they are another key to higher production because they save time. The use of route cards, route slips, route boards, light systems, and personal radios are all tools to consider. An increase in communication speed and accuracy ensures higher patient satisfaction, fewer mistakes, and greater profits.

"Liken your team to a symphony orchestra," said Alex. "There is one conductor and many players, each coming to the fore as the score dictates. When it all comes together, it's a thing of beauty."

Chapter 8

THE LOCAL DENTIST, DR. JACK MUDD

Not every dentist Alex came in contact with jumped at the chance to ask questions or come under his guidance. Dentists may feel threatened by competitors. They don't want to share why they are not doing as well as their neighbor. They don't want to share the methods and secret sauces that have led to their success. The neighborhood dentist you never hear from is most likely intimidated by you. When you never see them at CE (continuing education) courses, you wonder if they are keeping up with their skills. When you don't see them marketing, it gives you the impression that they are happy being small. When there is no expansion plan, it's obvious they intend to stay a solo practice. When you see team members leaving their practice and applying to work at yours, you know there are issues.

That was how Jack and Alex cohabitated in their small town. They were not close and knew little about one another. Dr. Mudd never thought to ask Alex how his practice was doing. At the Gwinnett Study Club quarterly meeting, Alex had a chance to chat with Jack, and after discussing the weather, the local high school sports team, and the state of the economy, the talk turned to dentistry.

Alex asked, "What do you worry about, Jack?"

Jack admitted, "My team is just not where I want them to be."

It turned out Jack was a loner, a do-it-yourselfer, not a delegator or leader. Crew members who could do it all, without him telling them what to do, were his best weapon, and he had few weapons on board.

"What makes you happy, Jack?" Alex asked. He knew the answers to a lot of Jack's questions but Jack would have to make the first move.

COMMITMENT TO CE, TRAINING, & MOTIVATION

Alex's questions about worry and happiness opened a communication between Alex and Jack. Jack came from left field sometimes, but at least he began asking questions.

"Why do I need to go to CE courses at this point in my career?" asked Jack.

"As dentists, we have an obligation to be continual students," said Alex, "but beyond ethical and legal obligations, we should stay on the leading edge of knowledge so that we keep our internal fires burning. Nothing stimulates more than being among forward-thinking, dynamic, eager dentists who want to share, learn, and do better. Excitement about what is better, new, or different stimulates and motivates us to achieve better outcomes for our patients. There is always a place for more CE, conferences, advanced training, dental masterminds, and online courses, no matter how long we have practiced dentistry. CE has been credited with bringing a number of drifting, burned-out dentists out of their funk, turning them back into the dynamos they once were.

"Are you looking to break out of your funk? Then it's time to jump into a new area of dentistry. Push the CE envelope. Maybe it's time you became the decathlon dentist in your town. Many times, a tired, ready-to-retire dentist has taken an advanced CE course, like the AAID maxi-course in implants, and totally reenergized his practice and his life. You can tackle dental aspects of sleep disorders. While many elements of dental practice require high degrees of manual dexterity and skill, making appliances for sleep apnea and snoring do not. Yet, those devices do require specialized understanding and knowledge. Spending a few years developing a sleep dentistry practice can be a less stressful and more lucrative way to finish well."

WEB-CENTRIC MARKETING GOING MOBILE

Some dentists know marketing, but most don't. Many dentists see what comes in the mail and think that is the sum total of marketing.

Jack did not do much marketing. He asked, "What good does marketing do when all you see are $29 exams and $600 crowns advertised? No dentist can make a profit on those fees."

Alex explained the roles of a loss leader, a call to action, and an irresistible offer to Jack and then said, "Jack, in ancient days, all roads led to Rome. Today, all roads, blogs, tweets, posts, and shares should lead to your website. WebCentric marketing means that the practice's website is the center of all your marketing efforts. Your website is the marketing hub, the center of all that is important about the practice. It is the place all patients should be directed in any form of marketing you do. If you want to succeed, three key ingredients need to be included in your WebCentric marketing action plan:

1. Mobile responsive
2. An irresistible offer
3. A strong call to action

"Meeting people where they are and how they interface with digital content is critical to getting eyes on your message. Hence, mobile responsive capability is necessary. The practice that does not plan for mobile use will lose market shares over time to those that do. To move people from spectator to customer, there needs to be a strong reason to make a choice. Give people your best offer, and they will respond. What do you find irresistible? Chances are others will feel the same way. When they do, they will buy.

"Everyone likes a deal, so get good at closing deals, but not all deals need to involve a huge discount. Added value often trumps discounts. Many people want access to a limited supply of a doctor's time. Many value the VIP status that comes with being an insider. How can you create added value without devaluing your services and decreasing your profitability? To cut the fee or not – that is the question! Do research and see how much more you will grow if you have a marketing action plan that includes some discounts for specific purposes. Those purposes could be filling hard-to-fill appointment slots, gaining new patients, reactivating patients who have not been in for several years, or filling in an empty schedule today. Another opportunity is when you have a new associate and need to fill their schedule. Anything is better than nothing because experience is gained, introductions are made, and referrals can result."

CROSS-TRAIN

Jack began to understand marketing and why fees were often discounted. It was foreign to him, but he was learning. As they talked, the topic turned to the additional work that would have to be done to implement some of the ideas Alex brought up.

Jack said, "I'm worried my staff will leave if I ask them to do one more thing. How do I deal with that fear?"

"Leadership creates a unifying vision that the entire team rallies around and focuses on achieving. Goals are set and achieved by the team. When the team's focus is on the purpose and not on themselves and how much they have to do, the practice will flourish. Team members need to know that they can get help whenever they need it. When one member is overloaded and stressed, there needs to be a mechanism for release.

"Only when team members are adequately cross-trained can that goal become a reality. Cross-training is the key to your success. In a small, one-doctor, three-staff member practice, it's essential that each knows how to cross over and do as much of another's job as legally allowable. The ability to make appointments, explain insurance, assist in a crown prep, make temps, coronal polish, and take X-rays is vital for all four (even the dentist) to know and do as needed.

"The larger the team, the more specialized job descriptions become. This is especially so with multi-doctor practices. Herein lays the challenge. Business assistants become isolated into HR, insurance, reception, or appointment scheduling and don't always have the training to assist dentists or take an FMX. Hygienists may be unable to clinically assist. As the team grows, without a cross-training plan, it becomes easier for team members to say, 'That's not my job.'

"More tasks will get done if there is no need to stop production and stop conversations with patients to find someone who can do a particular task. When the production line is held up by one broken gear in the entire system, the plant loses money. Similarly, in a dental practice, when the flow of the day has to halt to find Suzy, who is the only one who can take an accurate CT scan, the system is broken. So what is the big take-away here?" asked Alex. "Great teams cross-train and never have to hear, 'I don't know how to do that.'"

CONVERSIONS

Jack was listening and getting interested. His next question was more in tune with what would impact his practice.

"I'm not really good at selling dentistry, so how can I get my team to do it for me?"

"Another key aspect of attitude is the concept of 'team,'" Alex replied. "Dentistry is a partnership between all members of the team. To build for today, every team member should focus on filling every other team member's schedule for productive procedures. Imagine the synergy if five, ten, or fifteen team members were focused on filling your daily schedule.

"Conversions are all about moving a patient from one position to another, up the ladder of treatment. That might look like turning a phone call into an appointment or taking a new patient exam and turning it also into a productive same-day treatment with the dentist. A patient with a dental hygiene re-care appointment may be converted to include treatment with the doctor that same day after their hygiene visit. And vice versa, a restorative patient could move into an open hygiene operatory after their restorative appointment. Any time an opening occurs in the schedule, it is the team's job to announce it, recognize it, and fill it.

"How many times does a patient wish to start perio treatment after their consultation with the patient treatment coordinator? We don't know until we ask. When a patient is in the office getting a crown prep done and the schedule falls apart, have you ever offered to extend the current patient's appointment and work in three quadrants, not just one? How are your communication skills? A script is simply a set of lines that fit into a conversation where appropriate. Scripts are used most commonly to answer questions that patients ask. They may also be useful in sales and conversions, as in this conversation. If you have scripts and have practiced them, your team can convert many times a day when the need arises.

"Conversions strike at the most costly of all overhead items: broken and failed appointments. Conversions often save the day and create massive profit. If you consider conversions a good thing, you can pass average and become a superior practice. Most of my doctors in my masterminds become $10,000-a-day dentists because they have learned how to convert, and so have their team members. Conversions occur because of superior communication and well delivered spiels. Remember, if you ask a patient to do something, there is a 33% better chance of them saying yes if there is a 'because' following the request. People respond to requests at higher rates when reason is attached.

"A good example of a 'because statement' would be, 'Mrs. Jones, this tooth is in need of a crown to keep it safe and pain-free because there is a fracture running across the top and down the side of that molar, which could allow the cusp to break off and expose the nerve just from eating on it.' The *because* at the end gives the reason for the decision to be made. And so our key take-away today," said Alex, "is this: The team that converts well always hits or surpasses their goal."

Chapter 9

Alex's First Dream: The Walled City

Earlier, I said that success is, among other things, partly related to your dreams. Six to eight hours of every day are spent in sleep. Sleep is composed of three stages of non-REM sleep and one stage of REM sleep. A lot of things happen physiologically and mentally during sleep, including dreams. The purpose of dreams is not clearly understood, but Dr. Deirdre Barrett, a psychologist from Harvard University, postulates that one purpose of dreams is to solve two types of problems – those that require individuals to visualize something new, as an inventor of a new process or device, and those where "conventional wisdom is just wrong about how to approach a problem." She implies that a spark of intelligence is delivered to individuals during dreams. They receive inspired thought from out of the blue. Dreamers receive unexplained revelations in order to solve problems with which the mind is wrestling.

Understanding your dreams may provide insight into your own self and be a means of self-exploration, a key to unlocking your potential. Your dreams have the power to unify the mind, body, and spirit so that you can move forward in a more powerful way. When there is unity with your divine creator in your purpose, there is dunamis power on your side. Let's dig deeper into this divine connection and dunamis power.

The biblical rationale for studying your dreams

Consider the following scriptures:

"In the last days, God says, I will pour out my Spirit on all people. Your sons and daughters will prophesy, your young men will see visions, your old men will dream dreams." Acts 2:17 (NIV)

This is the prophetic message for those that hear in Acts and Joel 2:28, respectively. The Bible declares, in Psalms 16:7, that God counsels us at night through our dreams. Job 33:14-16 (NLT) gives further confirmation about God communicating with us via dreams. "For God speaks again and again, though people do not recognize it. He speaks in dreams, in visions of the night, when deep sleep falls on people as they lie in their beds. He whispers in their ears…"

How should you engage your dreams? Not all dreams are from God. How do you distinguish between them? Here is a five-step approach to dreams that will help you unlock their meaning and importance. First, pray that God will expose the source of the dream and give you meaning and insights as to what he wants to teach you through it. Second, listen to God, taking time to meditate before him so that you can hear more and get his perspective on the dream. When the peace of the Lord falls upon you and the presence of the Holy Spirit is felt, the communication will be clearer. Your spirit man will know when it is a supernatural encounter. Third, write your dream down so that you will not forget it. Time may pass before the meaning becomes clear. Fourth, seek godly counsel by sharing your dream with someone of wisdom. Be careful to not look for this wisdom in the wrong places. The spiritual world has two opposing sides and the counselor needs to be inspired and guided by the Holy Spirit. Fifth, let it be. God will cause his dreams to return to you, especially those that are most important. Rest in his presence and listen for his voice.

Alex and the Dream

"I looked and I saw a walled city," reflected Alex. "Around the central city, surrounded by a wall, four other walls extended to the North, South, East, and West. The people of the city were cut off from one another and spoke different languages. The customs, costumes, and cuisine of each reflected longstanding devotion to their ways."

Alex interpreted the dream to mean that dentists live isolated lives and often never talk to other dentists. They are like silos, which stand out as lone towers in the countryside. Those that go it alone are mentally miles apart from others and are thus called "silo dentists."

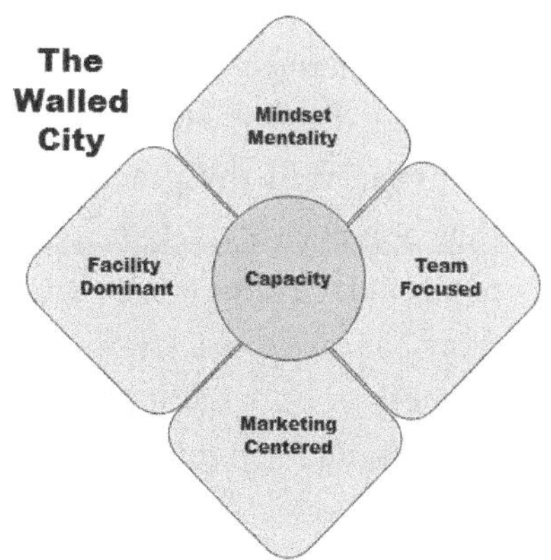

The city, divided into a central core and four quadrants, each separated from one another, alludes to five islands of thought in dentistry. One outer quadrant was dominated by Mindset Mentality, another was Team-Focused, the next appeared as Facility Dominant, and the last outer district was Marketing Centered. The older inner section of the city was Capacity. Alex had relocated into a new section of the city every decade and now in his fifth decade was living in the old part of the city, Capacity.

Silo dentists build walls around themselves and live separate lives. They may advance in some areas, but never put all the pieces together. Alex knew it was time to break down some of the walls, turn one-way streets into thoroughfares, and open the inner gates to restore communication between the inhabitants of the city. Alex described the city dream to those he came to tutor and gave them the key to one or more gates of the city so that they might move about more freely. Freedom is a wonderful thing.

To Dr. Blair Bennett, the young dental associate, Alex gave the key of "Willingness" because having the right mindset paves the way for an outstanding career.

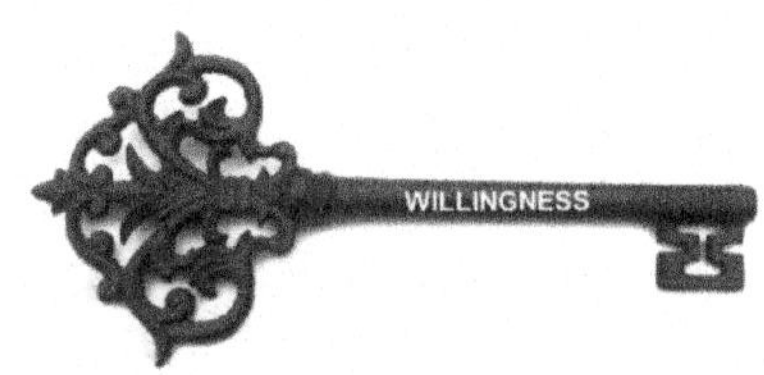

100% WILLINGNESS - GREAT ATTITUDE

You know the old saying. "Hire for attitude and train for aptitude." In dentistry, we can train the technical skills. That means bringing people on board who have a servant heart and a willing spirit. You want staff who believe in giving their best at all times – you want tens. Having tens at every position in the practice is a luxury many dentists desire, yet few achieve. Most tens are found rough, and then polished to perfection on the job in the crucible of the well-oiled dental practice. You must seek them, testing for attitude and willingness to do what it takes to be successful.

Willingness separates the average performer from the truly outstanding one. "I can" advances the cause so much more than "It's not my job." When a team member is willing to go the extra mile for you, you are willing to go the extra mile for them. Trust is developed; relationships are cemented. Loyalty is birthed, and the practice grows stronger and more capable. Remember, "Hire for attitude and train for aptitude."

To Dr. Edward Boyle, the servant dentist, Alex gave the key called "Time," so he could continue his mission work at home and abroad.

ELIMINATE WASTED TIME

We have eight hours in a typical work day. How do some dentists produce twice as much in that time as others? Could you see yourself working half as many hours making the same income or working the same hours as now but earning twice as much? The difference between a $10,000-a-day dentist and a $5,000-a-day dentist may be a matter of not wasting time!

When do you arrive at work? Are you ready to rock and roll at eight AM? Do you have an eight-at-eight or three-in-three mindset? Does your team share your penchant for being on time and efficient? Do you insist on your team preplanning, being on time, and filling up all available time on your schedule? After all, it is a mindset. Your capacity to produce a lot of dentistry is related to how you value and protect your time. A doctor's time is valuable and should be protected.

Delegation of non-essential duties creates time to be more productive. Effectively marketing for higher-end services provides the opportunity to be highly productive. Keeping a patient for longer, well-planned appointments is far more productive than ten smaller appointments.

So the big take-away today is this: increase your capacity by reducing wasted time. When you have more capacity, you buy back your time.

To Dr. Carley Matthews, the peak performer dentist, Alex gave the key called "Maximize," because she had the tools to know what to do with it.

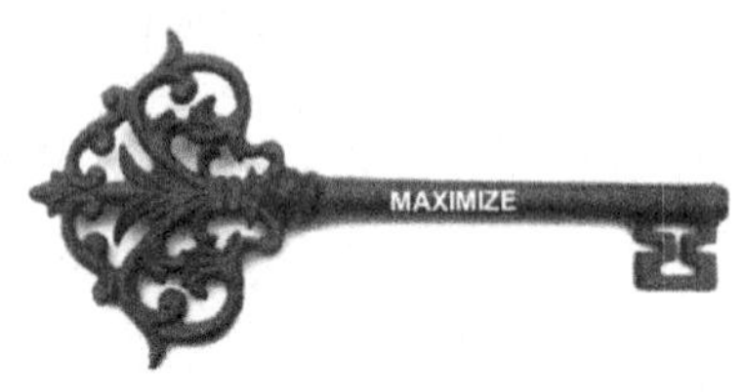

MAXIMIZE PATIENT REFERRALS

Fifty percent of new patients in a mature practice should come from direct patient referrals. A healthy practice replicates by having an open, welcoming front door and a protected, closed back door. When patients are happy and perceive value, they refer friends and family. When they feel pressured or cheated, they leave. Somewhere in between, they do nothing. They don't leave, but they don't refer. Increasing service and gaining better rapport will shift the needle to a more favorable position. How do you maximize your patient referrals?

- Ask. If you don't have, it's because you haven't asked. Give two business cards to patients at the end of an appointment—one for a friend and one for them.
- Care-to-Share cards that offer a deal for a friend and for the sharing patient are a great.
- Put up signs in the office saying, "We are accepting new patients."
- Have team bonuses for giving out Viva cards to patients so that they refer friends and family. Viva cards are like Care-to-Share cards, except they also have a magnetic strip to allow tracking the source of the cards when they are redeemed.
- Have games on Facebook that raffle prizes to those who share and like your Facebook page.

- The most certain way of getting patient referrals is to keep your current patients thrilled by being a gentle, on-time, painless dentist and thanking them for every visit, each referral, and each treatment they receive in your practice.

The most stable practices have most of their new patients referred by current patients. That is a worthy goal. Don't be afraid to ask your patients for referrals. The worst that can happen is that they say no, and if they do, you know you have something to fix.

The Maximize key is given to help you take advantage of the opportunity before you. Understanding your options will allow you to maximize your practice.

To Dr. Steve Blake, the mature dentist, Alex gave the key called "Flow," because with experience and a good practice, increasing patient flow through the system means dramatically higher profits.

FLOW

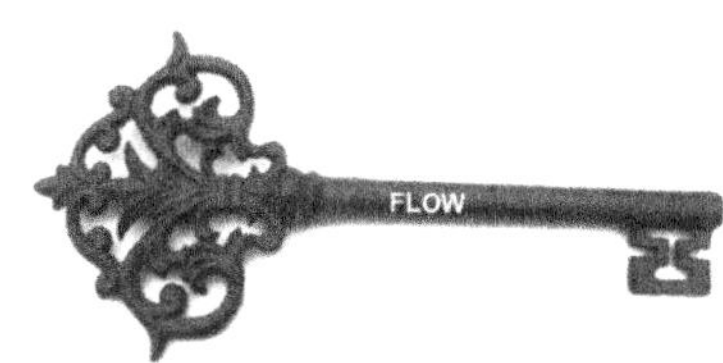

Patient flow through the practice is a big predictor of success. How productive a dentist is will often depend, in part, on how many rooms and clinical assistants are available to facilitate a high flow rate. With the mindset of abundance, willingness, readiness, and efficiency, a dentist can operate in three or four rooms (exclusive of hygiene rooms) with exceptional effectiveness.

To maximize potential, Alex recommends three or four clinical assistants per dentist working in three rooms, with one additional overflow operatory. While each clinical assistant should be cross-trained, one will always be the leader in ortho and TMD, one the leader in crown and bridge and one the leader in implants. You should focus on three major services for 75% of your production.

"In my own practice," Alex explains, "internal KPI for clinical assistants per dentist is one clinical assistant per $50,000 of production per month. Once you pass $50,000, hire an additional assistant. Once you pass $100,000 of production a month, add another."

Here's the take-away related to Flow: Don't let bottlenecks in your practice hinge on enough support to move willing patients through the system. Marketing is difficult and expensive; it's considered an investment. Don't waste money by marketing heavily if you are trying to save money by having a bare-bones team. Invest in good clinical assistants and they will pay their way time and time again.

To Dr. Jack Mudd, the local dentist, he gave the key called "Focus."

PATIENT-FOCUS – NOT SELF-FOCUS

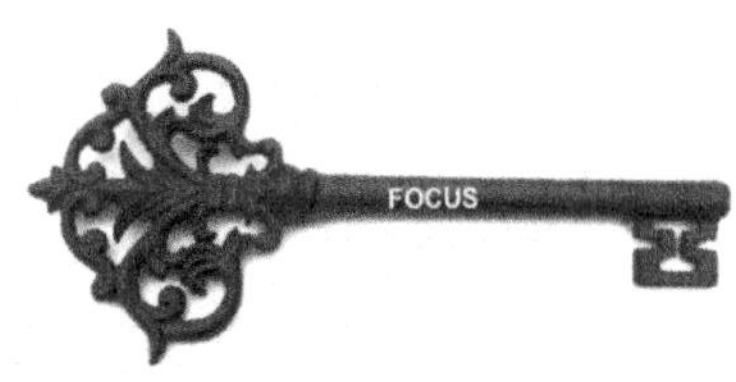

The tale of two dentists takes us to Focus Road. One dentist took the road called Self, and the other dentist took the road called Patients. The path to success on the self-focus road is long and winding, full of dangerous curves and sheer cliffs. The road to success on the patient-focus road, is wide, well-maintained, brightly lit, and lets us travel quickly and safely to our destination.

Dr. Dick Barnes teaches us to be firm in principle and flexible in procedure. Keeping patients happy is of utmost importance. Bend a little and gain a lot. Human nature is to fight for every little crumb and take advantage when opportunity knocks, even when it may hurt others. That point is vital to learning to be flexible and focused on others, not self. Awareness is the beginning of coming into a paradigm shift.

Dr. Marvin Belin shows how by saying yes and focusing on benefits to patients in our communications we can double our daily production. By being agreeable, we can get more of what we want. Interestingly, many dentists don't know how valuable time is to their patients. Just asking a few questions can lead to more dentistry in a day. If a patient really wants a big procedure done, your one-hour lunch isn't a necessity. Or if your home schedule is flexible and a support team is available, then just because it's 5:00 o'clock somewhere, that doesn't mean everyone has to go home.

The previous discussion about the "Say Yes" campaign expanded upon breaking through barriers that kept people from moving forward with needed dental care. Saving patients' time is one example. Saving the team time by not requiring the patient come back for exams and consults can add to the savings and boost the bottom line. This makes a practice more patient-focused, thereby increasing production. Doctors who are focused on improving practice finances will find that all team training on patient-focus will be among the highest ROI of any investment they make. One can be altruistic and still make a good profit.

Having a servant mindset means being patient-focused, meeting the needs of your patients, being flexible, and saying yes as often as you can. As my wife Sheila always says, "Take care of the patient and the money comes."

What Does Alex's Dream Mean for You?

In the end, the walls come down as our five dentists migrate from one section of the city to another, learning and growing to a new paradigm, a new way of understanding the practice of dentistry. Breaking free of limitations by adopting a new mindset will pay dividends over a career. The difference is that they are now comfortable moving between the city sections, and they enjoy the benefits of knowing all that there is to know and experience. It's only when dentists leave the nest and circle above the walls that they begin to see the infinite possibilities. Are you seeing the possibilities yet? The city represents the Big Five in dentistry – focus points that lead to a highly productive practice: Mindset, Team, Facility, Marketing, and Capacity.

When a dentist leads his or her team through the doors of opportunity, there is growth and comradery, something that cannot be measured but results in improvement and more stress-free days. Beginning with a facility strategy and implementing it gives every dentist a leg up on the competition. If patient flow is there through selective marketing, profitability can be achieved with proper training and financial systems.

As a dentist and his or her team gains maturity, symbolized by movement and growth within each city section, they eventually reach the pinnacle of their professional lives and arrive at Capacity, that place where capability and experience lead to increased capacity to build, manage, and enjoy their peak performing practice.

Chapter 10

ALEX'S SECOND DREAM: THE PARK

"If you will build it, he will come." In *Field of Dreams*, a mysterious voice comes to Ray (Kevin Costner). Alex heard a similar message. "It's time to build a better one," said the voice in his dream, referring to an adventure park where dentists and their teams take exhilarating rides and experience new ways of thinking as they evolve from average to extraordinary. Alex imagined a model of practice that was often dreamt yet seldom achieved. In Alex's dream, every man was an achiever. The banner over the entrance read: "Welcome to Opportunity Land."

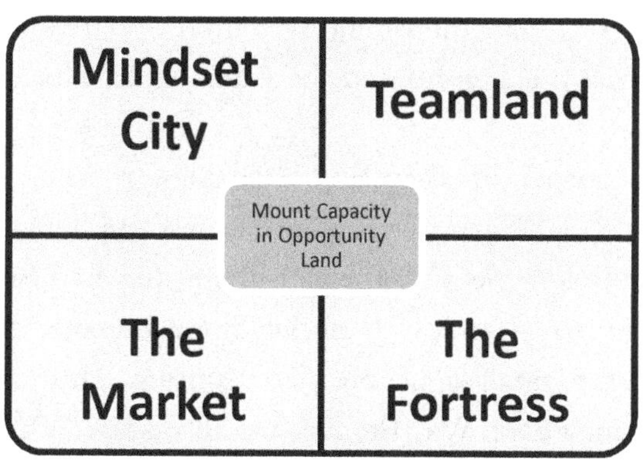

THE PARK

There were five sections to the park, just like the dream about the walled city. The grand entrance led to Mindset City and was the only gate into the park. It reminded Alex of Epcot Center, with grand overlays of Wolfgang Mozart and Johann Strauss playing in the background. In Possibility Exhibit Hall was a poster quoting Dr. Omer K. Reed. "If it's been done, it's probably possible." The Thinker Exhibit began with Napoléon Hill's timeless tome *Think and Grow Rich*. "Whatever the mind of man can conceive and believe, the mind can achieve."

The yellow brick road led guests to the next section of the park: Teamland. The door from Mindset City to Teamland was only four feet tall. Everyone had to bow low to enter. The message above the door into Teamland was James 4:10 (NIV). "Humble yourselves before the Lord, and he will lift you up."

The exhibit hall on the left had a giant LED screen that showed Alex's ideal team hard at work. Under the screen the caption read, "Teamwork Makes the Dream Work." Inside Teamland were adventure cruises to Jamaica, Cancun, skiing in Whistler, and a Hawaiian paradise. To the right was a dark Gothic building with the ominous warning, "There is no 'I' in TEAM." That building housed the Chamber of Horrors of lost teams.

In one corner of Teamland a small sign read, "Enter at Your Own Risk." There were many exits from Teamland, and many dentists left the park through them, finished for the day, going home to sleep on their accomplishments. But some teams saw the small sign and were curious. This rabbit hole must go somewhere. Was the risk worth taking? What was the payoff? Only a few took the chance to explore further. Rewards always come from risk.

The rabbit hole led through tunnels to the other side of the park. Opportunity knocks when one is curious and aware. The light at the end of the long tunnel became brighter, and the team entered a castle. As they emerged, they saw a sign welcoming them to The Fortress.

Most castles were of Romanesque design, sparse and austere, but this castle was ornate and in the baroque design of the Bavarian kings. It was not meant to fight wars but to celebrate success. This was the land of the kings and queens who built magnificent facilities to practice their craft. They built them and the people came.

One exhibit in The Fortress was named "Bigger Is Better." Another was called "A Horse in Every Stable." They saw "The Storehouse" and "The Vault." The team was surprised to find an exhibit in The Fortress titled, "Service above Self." What did service have to do with The Fortress? The only way to know was to enter and experience it. The way to success will sometimes take one to unexpected places and teach one unusual ways.

The inhabitants of The Fortress enjoyed their tour of the Banquet Hall. They were led past the demonstration kitchen, where they saw sumptuous meals being prepared. Then they sat at a long oak table in the banquet room to enjoy the lavish feast. The hall was filled with dancing, song, and merriment. At the end of the banquet, the Sargent at Arms rose and commanded, "Enter the Market. See from whence all these good things come." He opened the double doors into a garden, the next section of the park.

The Market was like nothing Alex had ever seen. He and his team stared in amazement at the neon lights and banks of video displays. It was like downtown Tokyo, Times Square, and Piccadilly Circus all rolled into one. Exotic sounds and smells embraced their senses. It was the sensorial experience of a lifetime. The Market was unlike any other place they had been. It wasn't what dentists usually did and it seemed foreign. There were many more exhibits here than in any other section of Opportunity Land. PR, the Social Six, Mailbox, the Seven Mountains, WebCentric, Radio, TV, Walkabout, and Niches each sounded promising. There was a carnival atmosphere, and barkers called to the people in the streets to come inside and see the show.

The exhibits housed the history of marketing through the ages and chronicled how dentists came to expand their marketing capability in 1978. The barkers called to passersby to come inside, learn, and experience that which was currently working. The value of marketing was clear. The purpose made sense, once it was explained.

At the end of the yellow brick road was a door called "Just Do It." It was the only door, the only exit on the street, unless one wanted to retrace one's steps and return to formerly visited sections. Alex and the others opened "Just Do It," stepped inside and were transported to the peak of Mount Capacity. From there, they realized that they could see farther and understand more than they had ever known. The messages from the other exhibits began to make sense. Ten displays ringed the summit, and each revealed how the masters achieved excellence and perfection. As they passed through, the final keys to success were handed to those dentists and teams who had continued steadfastly and purposefully through the park. Their persistence had led them to the top of Mount Capacity, where they finally rested. They had come into the Land of Opportunity.

Carley's Key

Alex understood the keys and knew who among his protégés could use those most. Because of Dr. Carley

Matthew's well-developed skillset and growing reputation, clients came to her asking for treatment. She needed to be more efficient to become more productive. To create more capacity, Alex handed her the "Multiples" key.

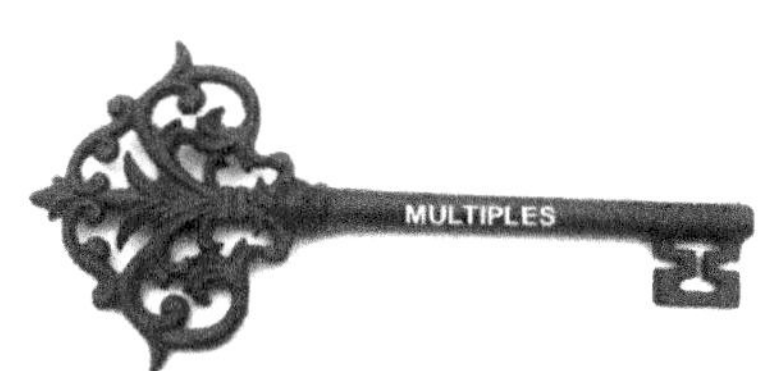

MULTIPLE DISCIPLINES PER APPOINTMENT

The decathlon dentist is in the catbird seat when it comes to scheduling and maximizing capacity. Because you understand how to treat everything you diagnose, you can structure a patient's treatment to meet (1) their time requirements, (2) their apprehension or fear factor level, (3) their financial capacity, and (4) your own schedule. You can do everything in one day or over five years. You can do endo, extractions, perio, and restorative all in one appointment with one injection for the quadrant, or you can bring them in for all their treatment needs, employing five or six different dental disciplines in the same appointment.

"I've had many patients tell me that another dentist said they couldn't be numbed on both sides of their mouth, but we do it every day," explained Alex. "Combining more dentistry per appointment is wise. Leave dental school thinking behind. Combining multiple procedures is especially attractive to dental-phobes when sedation dentistry is planned and utilized." Patients love a dentist who thinks like a patient and just gets it done!

A Key for Blair

Alex's keys from the top of Mount Capacity in Opportunity Land clinked on their metal ring. Which key would best fit Dr. Blair Bennet and her practice as an associate in his own office? Her successful progress would benefit the practice he owned, so it was a win-win situation to help her grow her practice rapidly. That was the goal – fast but solid, steady growth. For that reason, Alex advised Blair to become a pillar in the community. He told her about "Walkabout."

WALKABOUT

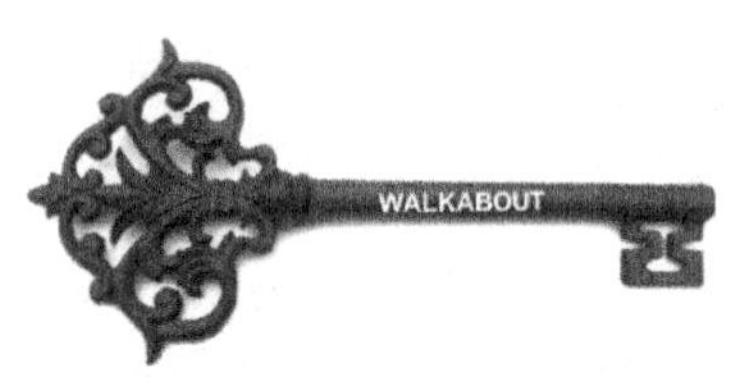

When a young aborigine in Australia came of age, he went on a trek through the wilderness called a walkabout. This was a time of leaving the nest, a test of skill and courage on the way to becoming a man. Today, a dentist leaves school and the comfort of educational confines starts out in their new career. "Walkabout" is a key ingredient to early practice success.

You're new and no one knows you. You have no friends, no reputation, and no allies. One of the first activities Alex recommends to a new dentist is a walkabout. Get out and meet the business owners, clerks, professionals, and people of influence in the area. Put shoe leather to the sidewalk and engage with the community. Get to know them before you ask them to become your patients.

Create a public relations campaign and run it prior to beginning your walkabout. Have your marketing message and materials in place, and in hand, before your walkabout. Then, when the time is right, you'll have something to hand to those you meet. Do something newsworthy every month to get your name out into the media. Walk door-to-door, meeting and greeting your neighbors. Walkabout is one segment of your Authority Marketing Strategy, helping you become the local expert. To be seen as an expert, you have to invest time and energy and put yourself out there where people can see you, talk to you, and gain trust in who you are. To become a force in business, you have to force yourself to Walkabout.

The Mudd Key

Alex had seen the face of Dr. Jack Mudd's practice. He had not updated it in many years, so the first move Alex suggest was a makeover of the facility. The key to improvement was one everyone would notice.

CURB APPEAL

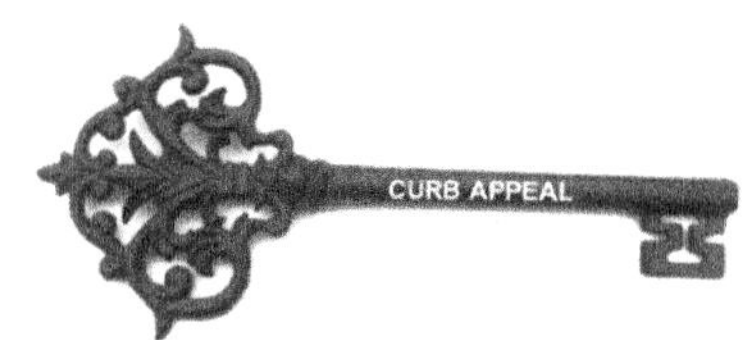

Did you ever pull up to the curb of a classy restaurant and have the valet attendant open your door and invite you in for a fine dining experience? Your expectations are through the roof as you enter the facility, and you hope the maître d', the servers, and chef do not disappoint. Great curb appeal whets the appetite for what will happen inside. Curb appeal is all about setting expectations.

What your patients perceive from the outside carries the same weight. Setting and meeting expectations is the name of the game for the $10,000-a-day dentist. To become one, you must appear to be one. Discriminating individuals expect their dentists to be successful. It's okay to park your Jaguar in the front parking lot. It's okay to have an artwork-filled reception area. The exterior and interior are a statement, a sign of who you are and what values you hold.

Speaking of signs, the most cost effective advertising you will ever do is your signage. Take special care to have it say who you are in eye-catching, colorful, tastefully-done, brightly-lit elegance. The grass and shrubs around your building need to be trimmed regularly, just like your own haircut. Lighting should be more than adequate; it should be dramatic, enhancing the property and focal points, not simply illuminating. To attract the influential and the affluent, you must have curb appeal.

Edward's Key to Door Number Three

Every dentist has a worldview under which they operate. Some choose Door #1, where it's all about building a solid family supported by a well-run dental practice. Behind Door #2 is the entrepreneur. Build it big and make an impact. Edward Boyle was more of a Door #3-type dentist; he chose to serve his patients to the fullest extent and to serve those who were less able to help themselves. When you have experience, skills, and places to go and things to do other than your dental practice, you need to be more efficient with your time and energy. That's what Alex wanted to impart to Dr. Edward Boyle. Being a real servant, going on missions, and working at the local Good Samaritan Health Center, Edward would be better able to serve both of his passions by delegating tasks to his new patient coordinator.

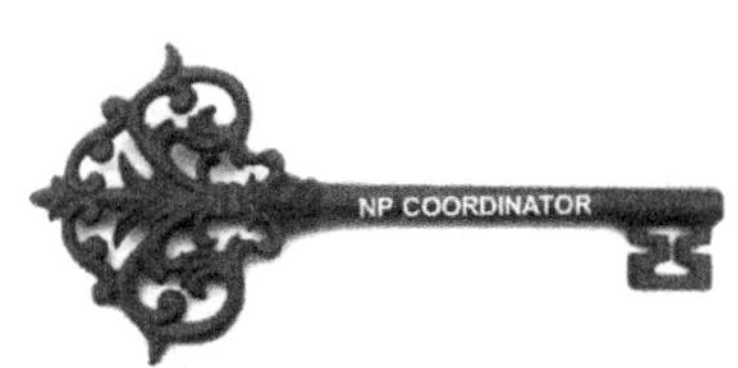

NEW PATIENT COORDINATOR

How do you feel when you are escorted to a hotel room by a bellman that draws the drapes, shows off the amenities and the minibar, demonstrates how to operate the safe in the room, and asks if there are any questions before he leaves? The new patient coordinator fills the same role. They take a new patient on a tour of the office before the dental staff goes on a tour of his or her mouth. The NPC shows new patients the layout of the facility, introducing them to each team member they encounter, explains the photos, diplomas, certificates, and mission memorabilia on the walls as well as the purpose of each major piece of equipment.

The new patient coordinator escorts the patient into the interview room and reviews the paperwork, including medical and dental history. She completes the initial interview with the patient, learns their "hot buttons" and the primary reason for their visit. It is the beginning of the bonding process and establishes rapport and trust. The NPC shows the new patient gratitude for coming to the practice, educates the patient on who you are, and empathizes with their concerns. Once all the important information is gathered, the doctor is given a summary by the NPC away from the new patient, before their formal meeting with the dentist.

This system allows for maximum flexibility of the doctor's schedule and makes it possible for the dentist to arrive at the meeting with a new patient primed and ready to conduct the perfect initial interview.

The Key That Set Steve Free

Dr. Steve Blake knew nothing about "spa dentistry," but Alex thought he should. As the elder dentist in town, Steve already had status and authority over his rivals. What he needed was a story that would start a buzz around town.

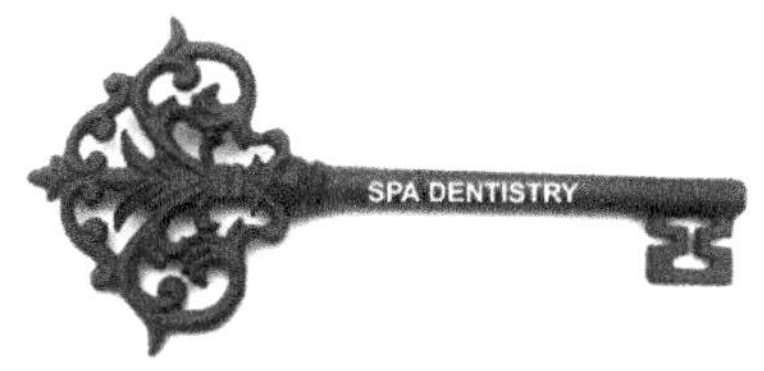

SPA DENTISTRY

The big push in the cosmetic boutique era was the dental spa. Catering to those who wanted a refined, upscale experience, the spa dentist offered massage chairs, aroma therapy, neck warmers, blankets, paraffin wax hand treatments, and soothing music. Alex took a leap and offered a special spa room that he called "The Resting

Room." There a patient could relax in cozy leather chairs under subdued lighting, browse on their iPhones, or sit at the Internet Café stations using one of the laptops provided. Patients were invited to "come early and stay late" after their dental appointments. It was an oasis, a sanctuary from the world, a place for patients to escape and enjoy a few minutes alone.

What separates your practice from the one down the street? Are you unique? What do your patients tell their friends about your practice? When you set yourself and your practice apart from all the rest, you become the one they talk about. You become the "celebrity dentist," the one that people call to endorse political candidates, be the team dentist for high school sports teams, or speak on dentistry at the Rotary Club. Having a resting room and a spa-like atmosphere can generate a buzz around town that leads to future benefits.

The big take-away: Make your practice something to talk about. Create a story that begs to be told. Marketing and public relations are meant to define you by telling a simple story of who you are and what you do.

Chapter 11

Alex's Third Dream: Land of the Vikings

Sometimes Alex had recurring dreams. That generally meant that they were significant, that they were a message for today. God's breath is imprinted on our DNA and he sometimes speaks to us and gives us inspiration through dreams. Through dreams Alex saw himself cruising the North Atlantic in centuries past on modern ocean liners. "What is the meaning?" he wondered. "And who are the people with me in my dream? Why am I dreaming of past and present?"

Northwestern winds caught and filled their sails, yet the Norsemen pulled on their oars to propel their ship out of the fjord toward the icy salt water of the North Sea, heading south to Scotland and England. Sailing into the unknown, searching for new lands and adventure – this was the allure of the sea. Alex was an adventurer and a romantic at heart. He sought escape from the ordinary. He often yearned to be at sea, seeking new lands and experiences, like the Norsemen. Such was the recurring dream that Alex shared with his protégés.

Not long afterwards, that dream became reality and the present journey began.

The Explorers Club

Melting aquamarine glacial waters spilled over two hundred-foot waterfalls into the deep blue water of Norway's Geirangerfjord. Every half hour or so, a crack like a rifle shot echoed in the fjord as the glacier lost tons of ice to the water below. Three thousand-foot granite walls soared above the *Viking Star*. Alex's dream of Viking expeditions to foreign lands came to fruition when he hosted the Explorers Club: Top Gun Conference at Sea aboard the Viking ocean cruiser. His conference had morphed from a meeting in his practice's teaching facility in Stone Mountain, Georgia, to the elegant Lake Lanier Islands resort and now a North Sea cruise from London to the Norwegian fjords. Continuing dental education in exotic places had always been a dream for Alex, and it had finally come true.

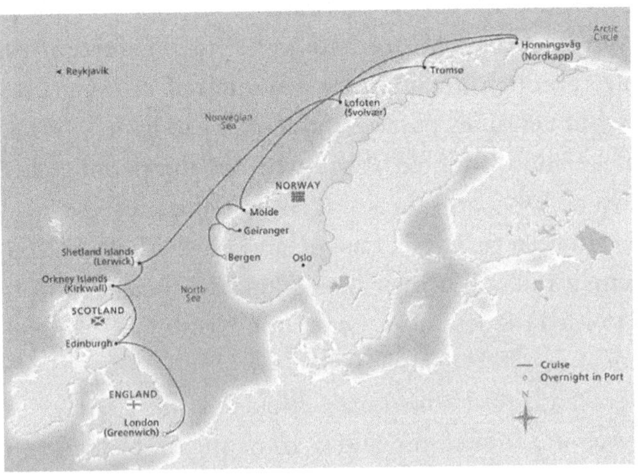

The Top Gun Conference at Sea Ports of Call

He chose Viking Ocean Cruises because they always did everything first-class. Alex's experience sailing the Yangzi in

China and the Rhine/ Main/ Danube Rivers across the heart of Europe with Viking proved them worthy of hosting a Top Gun Conference. Their recent interest in expanding into educational offerings meant that they were open-minded and seeking peak experiences for their clients.

The first days of the expedition were spent in vibrant London, England, where Alex gave the opening address to the Top Gun Conference. The theme of this conference was maximizing daily performance, and Alex drove that point home with his keynote lecture on KPI: What Gets Measured Gets Done.

KPI AND THE GOAL KEY LIST*

"What gets measured gets done." If you put critical elements and processes in logical, chronological order and accomplish each step before moving on, you will be successful. If you employ these two management principles, you will develop the mindset of the $10,000-a-day dentist and then, over time, actually become a highly productive dentist.

KPI, or *key performance indicators*, are the elements, numbers, and activities that move the needle forward. Your practice advances when you measure the performance of individuals, groups, and business processes. Copying what successful practices do and comparing your numbers to theirs gives you a meaningful yard stick by which to measure growth. That's why we use benchmarks and compare ourselves to other successful practices. We measure everything because everything is important.

During the lecture, Alex asked those who felt uncomfortable with numbers, spreadsheets, and graphs to raise their hand. Dr. Blair Bennett was among the first to admit that she did not get much business training in dental school and would not know the best measurements. Alex thought a well laid-out plan is one in which the end is known and the doctor works backwards from that end to achieve success. In essence, that is the message of the Gold Key List.*

*Author's Note: The Gold Key List is a list of one hundred tasks that I completed to grow my practice from zero to $5.8 million over ten years. It's the basis of the teaching in the 5M Masters Academy. Understand and complete the Gold Key List series of tasks, and create the practice of your dreams. Those who complete the Gold Key List are likely to be called $10,000-a-day dentists!

The Scottish Experience

The Explorers Club was on a roll. Edinburgh Castle towered above the harbor as the *Viking Star* lay at anchor. The evening educational program was delivered by Dr. Joe Ellis, Dean of the Solstice Research Group, an international study club twenty-seven years in existence. His topic was The new patient experience and patient flow. Joe explained it began in the Solstice Group and how it evolved over twenty years. His principal point was creating effective consults.

CONSULT ROOM

Give serious consideration to this room. Your consult room is where serious conversations occur. Nothing should happen there by accident. This room determines 95% of the success of your practice. You need your best person manning the position, and you need ideal surroundings to get the job done.

What makes the consult room effective? First, you need certificates and signs of your expertise and authority on the walls. Second, you need a room behind etched-glass doors that provides a quiet, private space but allows the team to know when the patient treatment coordinator is busy. Models, charts, diagrams, and videos for every possible treatment should be readily available to show patients. A printed, organized treatment plan personalized for each patient should be ready. A consultation folder for the patient to take home is prepared with all details, including intra oral photographs of existing failing dentistry as well as the solution to those problems. When doing a treatment plan presentation, preparation is the most important ingredient. Have your ducks in a row. Know your scripts and be able to handle objections.

It's not always the patient who needs to be present at the treatment plan presentation. A chair for significant others who help make financial decisions that affect the family is important and should be filled on a regular basis. Explaining it in detail to the person who makes financial decisions is far more important than most realize. If you don't set up the consultation with the right person, a lot is lost in translation, including—often—your entire case!

Dr. Joe Ellis's lecture on patient flow, the proper use of the consult room, and how the PTC fills the need to delegate duties was a favorite of the dentists, especially Dr. Jack Mudd. He liked having his team be the ones to sell the dentistry. He understood that the key to good case acceptance was a great new patient experience with a team member. Selling dentistry stresses some dentists and they show that stress on their faces, in their voices, and in the answers they give to questions. When a patient senses stress, their confidence wanes and case acceptance suffers. Selecting the right person to obtain treatment acceptance is critical. Let the dentists do what they do best—take care of their oral health needs. Jack knew he was not the best fit for selling dentistry. He was glad to delegate it to his office manager.

Another Day, another Island, another Lecture

SOCIAL PROOF

Into the North Sea and the windswept Shetland Islands and Outer Hebrides they sailed. Dr. Lee Ostler, founding member and past president of AAOSH, the American Academy for Oral Systemic Health and an original member of the Solstice Research Group, led the talks through the North Sea exploration. His expertise in dentistry was multifaceted and the focus this week was on Social Proof. His pivotal point to doctors was to show up early, often, and everywhere patients are likely to look.

What's on your walls? As a new patient is toured through the office they learn about you and your practice from the NPC and what's on your walls. You know about Social Proof and its value. A dentist needs to display why they are relevant, why they are the best choice for their dentist. Social Proof gives evidence of what others say, think, and believe. It takes impressions created by public relations and marketing ads and turns them into reality in a patient's mind. There are four places you need to show up.

1. Social Media and the Internet—the so-called new media. Posts on your "wall," likes and shares, pins and re-postings of your blog. Remember, this is an evolving media. Posting photographs are better than posting text, video is better than photos, and live streaming video is superior to all else.

2. Radio, TV, Print Media—these may be considered "old guard," but they are still highly trusted media. An effective motto is "Be seen and be seen often." Interviews are great, but having your own show tops everything. Those who dominate mainstream media also dominate the competition. Trust is higher when potential patients see you as an authority figure, and nothing screams authority more than a published book or a TV, radio, or magazine interview, except having your own radio or TV show. Dentists who are authors of books explaining how patients can have better smiles, improved health, and greater longevity are going to inspire trust in their patients.

3. On your office walls display before and after photos, testimonials, and reviews. All of this matters, whether it's on your office walls or on Yelp, Google, and, your practice's reviews page.

4. Word of mouth. Referrals from satisfied customers are the best kind of social proof and the reason mature practices need to spend half as much on marketing as young practices. Don't forget to have a MAP, a marketing action plan, to maximize marketing strategy in your practice.

Fifty percent of the mature practices' new patients come from word of mouth referrals. This is the ultimate goal of marketing – building a happy, stable, and referring patient base. Dr. Ostler reminded the attendees of the Top Gun Conference at Sea that all dentists need to maximize social proof for their practices. Social proof can tell a story. It is one of the most effective ways of marketing. When someone like Dr. Edward Boyle goes on a mission trip like the one he went on with Alex to Kenya, the community where Dr. Boyle practices needs to hear and read about it. By being proactive, you make it happen. The squeaky wheel gets oiled and the promoted practice gets noticed. When marketing your practice, it's important to be seen everywhere and be seen often.

The Expanding Concept

Bergen, the Nordic base of the Vikings, was the next port of call for the *Viking Star*. From there, Alex and his group began fjord-hopping, cruising deeper into the interior of the Norwegian homelands. Noted biological dentist Dr. Nicholas Meyer, author of *The Holistic Dental Matrix*, had been Alex's friend for years. When he was ready to slow down and think of retirement, he had not had sufficient assets. He had talked to Alex about a solution. They formulated a plan and within two years, Nick had brought in an associate dentist, and doubled and transitioned the practice. His nest egg was secured, and he did what he had dreamed of doing.

Bringing in an associate is critical to finishing well. A good transition only occurs when you plan ahead. Nick presided over the next series of Top Gun Lectures and gave the dentists the following charge: "Develop your expansion plan now."

EXPANSION PLAN

Robert Burns wrote, "The best laid schemes of mice and men often go awry." In Alex's plan to develop his new practice, he originally envisioned a three-operatory, three-day-a-week boutique cosmetic practice. Little did he know he would grow it into a fifteen-operatory, four-dentist, twenty-five-staff behemoth.

He accidently hit upon a golden idea—the expandable dental facility. The person who gets this one point will likely make a fortune. What one starts out with is rarely what one finishes with. If you could build the ideal facility for a solo practitioner and have it grow as your practice grows, that would be a plus. To choose one location, one facility, and not have to reinvent your practice every ten years would save hundreds of thousands, if not millions, in expenses and lost revenue. Imagine how many dollars have been lost starting over, moving because the facility did not work. What if you could start small and build as need and growth allowed? What if you could plan to have a group practice before you need it? Can you see where this is headed?

The big take-away is this: Build it with the end in mind. Build and lease expandable space with the option to buy. Get first right of refusal to occupy space as you grow and expand. Owning is better than renting. Having an associate to share the load, help grow the practice, and increase its value is a major part of the plan to finish well. Dentists who want to retire with a large nest egg do it by creating income centers. They invest in infrastructure and employ other dentists to create cash flow through the practice, increasing the net value of the practice. Economy of scale is maximized when multiple dentists operate in a single space, sharing overhead and expensive technology, such as cone beam CT, CEREC systems, and K7 neuromuscular systems.

When a practice is to be sold, the purchase price is based on two things: earnings and profits. To maximize your earnings, you need multiple hands on deck. To maximize your profits, you need efficient systems and a steady flow of patients. Alex knew that every dentist in the room would benefit from Dr. Meyer's advice, especially Dr. Steve Blake. He had five to ten more years to work if he wanted to, so the expansion plan could easily double his practice's value. Alex was proud to see that Nick had been so successful and was sharing his story with other dentists. Those were the rewards Alex enjoyed most.

The Cruise Continues

Sailing into the Land of the Midnight Sun above the Arctic Circle, the *Viking Star* reached Honningsvag. The last speaker on the voyage was Dr. Geoff Pratt, of Victoria, Canada. His topic was "Balance." Geoff was a charter member of the Solstice Research Group. He had moved from Guelf, Ontario, to Victoria as part of his plan to finish well before retiring. His career revolved around training at the Pankey Institute. Geoff's job was to put it all into perspective for the group.

BALANCE

Being a $10,000-a-day dentist is not all about making money and seeking maximum capacity. Money is just a way to measure service. Serving yourself must be in the equation, as well as serving your family, your community, and your God. Geoff's focus, ever since attending the Pankey Institute, had been to balance the Cross of Life: work, play, love, and spiritual.

Dr. Pankey's Cross of Life represented lifestyle equilibrium. What we put into life equals what we get out of life when all the parts are balanced. When they are out of balance, the overweighed segment drags down the other parts and places us in jeopardy of overload, which can lead to breakdown. Much of our effort should be put into planning our lives so that there is adequate input into each of the four quadrants of The Cross of Life.

We serve one at the expense of the other in some cases. We get unbalanced. But what if we could serve all at the same time? When we place our values properly centered on good, guiding principles, we violate none of the rules. When we give our best effort to our patients, when we follow God's Golden Rule, when we honor our family and spend adequate time at rest for ourselves, we bring balance to our lives. We have the awesome opportunity to live fruitful and balanced lives. Planning life is as important as planning a career, planning a year, or planning a patient's case. Plan balance in your life. It takes TIME.

Top Gun Balancing Act

Listening to Geoff's lecture on balance, Alex thought the lesson would be particularly well suited to Dr. Carley Matthews. Top Gunners often tend to be out of balance and need someone to call them back to center now and then. The role of mentor and coach is to do just that. The higher a dentist moves up the career ladder, the more potential stress there is upon them and the more visible they are. A coach can steady their climb upwards and assist the safe descent.

Dentists need time away from the grind. Being at the office all the time can be detrimental to physical, mental, and spiritual health. Balance is better than burning the candle on both ends.

Alex found international travel mixed with continuing education a refreshing change of pace that added to his knowledge and skills, as well as his sense of adventure. The next time you're looking for a break, consider an international dental getaway and include a few personal days for refreshing and decompressing.

Chapter 12

THE SILICON SANDBOX

The wisdom of the ages is stored on paper and silicon. The internet, with sites like Google, Project Gutenberg, and Wikipedia, means this wisdom is instantly available. Combined with LinkedIn and Facebook groups, we are all smarter together than we are as individuals. Artificial intelligence is in its infancy, but the answers to vital questions are at your fingertips. Along the way, Alex was posed five questions, one each from his five protégés. He referred them to Google, the king of the silicon sandbox, for an answer. Here are the results.

Dr. Blair Bennett asked, "Since I'm a relatively new dentist, how can I gain an edge over other dentists in my area? I don't have extensive experience, a track record to showcase, or a file of patients from whom to expect referrals. What will set me apart from other dentists?" She had latched onto an idea Alex called trumping. To trump one's competitor is to outsmart them. When you can do something that your competition can't do or offer a service your competition can't offer, you have an edge over them.

SEDATION DENTISTRY

Nothing will open the door to more new patients than sedation dentistry. Fully fifty percent of the populace actively avoids the dentist because they have anxiety and extreme dental phobia. They are one of the most underserved groups and they live and work in your community. Dental phobics have shut the door to dental visits.

If you offer patients nitrous oxide gas, you'll see a crack in the doorway. When you offer conscious sedation, what Alex calls "the pill," you'll swing the door half way open. By offering I.V. sedation, you swing the new patient door wide open. There are three good reasons to offer sedation dentistry beyond the obvious:

1. The cases you'll see are more involved because the phobic patient has put off treatment for such a long time. This type of treatment is usually more complex and rewarding for a dentist. Remember, the rewards in the dental arena are not just financial. Treating phobic patients is heart-warming. Our psychological need for love, acceptance, and helpfulness to others is satisfied.

2. These people commit to paying their fees in advance and get it all done in one or two visits. They don't want to be fully awake for any procedure, they don't want to remember being there, and they certainly don't want to come back ten or twenty times. There is efficiency in sedation dentistry that begs dentists to consider offering this service.

3. Phobic patients make the best referral patients because once treated they have such a dental "non-experience" to rave about to their friends. A dental practice cannot have too many enthusiastic, loyal, referring patients.

If you want to build your practice, go after the silent majority that sits on the sidelines and waits, and waits, and waits. They can be your secret to success.

The big question put to Google from Dr. Edward Boyle was, "What are the best social media platforms on which to share my stories?" There's nothing like asking a robot what robot to use to market your practice!

THE SOCIAL SIX

The marketing world was turned upside down when Google, Facebook, and YouTube entered the picture. Social media now dominates the discussion, and you need to capture your place in the Social Six. The Social Six are Google+, Facebook, YouTube, Twitter, Pinterest, and LinkedIn. Many will come and go, new platforms will challenge, like Instagram or SnapChat as of late, but for now, these are the six platforms on which you need to appear. Each of the six has a purpose and will secure for you a slice of the social media pie. Grow your presence on social media with advanced strategies, and your number of new patients will skyrocket.

Amateur actions deliver mediocre results. A professional approach to each social platform will bring superior results. Ride the waves of the Social Six and keep watch for the next social wave on the horizon.

Dr. Carley Matthews asked about technology. "What is the most important technology to improve production and profits?" Google would show her a word cloud for her answer.

TECHNOLOGY RULES

Yes, technology rules. When patients seek to differentiate one dentist from another, they often look to see what technology the practice embraces. Here is a list of the major technologies you may want to employ to achieve the highest standard of patient care and gain the greatest amount of influence with tech-savvy patients who truly care about these matters.

1. Dental lasers – Alex has five of them in his practice. Patients love lasers. Alex uses them every day for a variety of procedures and never fails to get comments from his patients about their use.
2. CAD-CAM optical scanners and immediate crown creation is increasingly important, a must-have tool for the future.
3. Digital radiology – Immediate, low dose images are state of the art for intra oral, panoramic, and cone beam CT. You need them now. More on CBCT later.
4. Digital photography and intra oral photography. The more you use these tools, the greater your case acceptance. They are critical to your success.
5. K7 – Biopack – EMG and TENS for diagnosis of TMD, pain, major reconstruction, and orthodontic cases. If you aspire to do a plethora of $30,000 and up cases, you'll need advanced training in handling alteration of existing occlusions, vertical dimensions, and mandibular relationships.
6. Diagnodent and Cariview for caries detection. Nothing is simpler into diagnose and easier to explain to patients as a conservative method of saving tooth structure. Alex uses these every day on every patient.
7. Velscope for oral cancer screening. If you save one life, the effort is worth it. My associate dentist Dr. Jeremy Smith's dad was diagnosed with throat cancer, which brought it home to us in a flash. We doubled our efforts to be proactive in oral cancer screening for every one of our patients. He survived because it was caught in time. We continue to poke, prod, and screen in hopes of saving another, just like Jeremy's dad.
8. Oral DNA testing for pathogenic periodontal bacteria. This is an integral part of our perio program. Having an oral-systemic connection discussion with every patient

leads to higher case acceptance and higher total case fees.

9. T-Scan for occlusal analysis and bite balancing. It's time to go beyond articulating paper blue marks to grind in the occlusion. This is the definitive way to know your occlusion is correct.
10. Trios*, Iterro, 3M Digital Impression Technology. The science and reliability of this process has advanced to the point that impression material is as unnecessary for many cases as is shipping a box to the lab. In many instances, digitizing information leads to increased efficiency, accuracy, and speed of case completion. Fewer remakes, better fits, reduced chair time, and less expensive restorations all benefit the patient, the laboratory, and the practice.

*Author's note: Since getting the Three Shape Trios optical scanner, I have used it to scan 98% of my cases, doing very few by PVS impression alone (on my two full-mouth cases I took a backup PVS impression). The lab received the cases five minutes after they were digitized and instructions sent via the silicon pathway. Best of all, of the cases returned from the lab (300+ units), we have had less than 1% remakes, and most of those were for color modifications. It's easy to see why labs love this digital technology. Dentists will, too!

CONE BEAM CT

One of the smartest business decisions you can make as a decathlon dentist is to buy a combination cone beam CT – panoral X-ray machine. Here's why:

1. Hygiene – You'll need panoramic film on all patients every four years. That's a lot of use and will help to pay for the machine in a brief amount of time.

2. Dental implants – CBCT is a state-of-the-art and standard-of-care issue and in my opinion, it is required to use a CBCT image for most every case. You'll double the number of implants placed when you know there is adequate bone. Undesirable sequelae are reduced by using high-tech solutions. Regarding dental implants, look into ceramic zirconia options for patients who want more biocompatibility and highly aesthetic results.
3. Oral surgery – third molars require panoramic films, but some impactions require a CT to know critical details like cysts, roots near nerves, sinus shape, and more.
4. The CBCT takes the most accurate TMD films, and airway problems can be diagnosed as well. CBCTs now help diagnose endodontic lesions and root systems, as well as endodontic failures, which are far more common than expected. 2D films are far from adequate in diagnosis of endodontically involved teeth.

Dedicate space in your facility for one combo cone beam CT-PAN machine and deliver the highest standard-of-care possible. Technology does not mean only hardware in the office. It can indicate software and outsourced services like Maccrony or OnFire Reviews. Using the technology of the day, whether it be DFY (done -for -you) services or innovative apps and software solutions, dental practices that embrace best practices will far exceed their competition.

The Big Take-Away: Technology rules!

Dr. Jack Mudd asked Google how to streamline his team positions. Google was in step with Alex on all counts. The answer that came up first was "Concierge."

CONCIERGE POSITION

The Supremes had it right. Their chart-topper in 1964 said it all. "Stop in the name of love, before you break my heart. Think it over."

When a new patient stops into your office for the first time, your team needs to "show them the love." This is best accomplished by having a true receptionist, what we call our dental concierge. Her job is to meet and greet all of our patients, direct their calls, sign them in, answer their questions, introduce them to the therapists they'll be working with that day, and, finally, bid them a warm goodbye after they have completed treatment. Show them your heart and they will be patients for life.

Concierges allow for fewer interruptions of appointment schedulers, insurance handlers, treatment coordinator, office manager, and collection and financing personnel. They deflect incoming traffic. Removing distractions from other team members is a key benefit of employing a dental concierge. They are the smiling face of the practice, and they get to love on patients all day long! When your practice reaches the ideal size, you'll want to consider the dental concierge as one essential "people person" position for your dental team. When interviewing for a dental concierge, look for smiling faces and warm hearts.

Dr. Steve Blake asked the $64,000 question, "What is the most important reason some dentists outperform others?" Many answers popped up, including having enough space (operatories or surgeries) to fully function in the most efficient manner.

NUMBER OF OPERATORIES

Having the right number of operatories allows a dentist to function efficiently and grow. Staying ahead of the growth curve is one key to building a successful practice and career. As an owner/ dentist grows the practice, associate dentists can be hired to help manage increasing patient numbers and allow time for the owner to work on the practice and take vacation and continuing education time away. Managing other dentists can dramatically enhance profit for the owner/ dentist.

It's not just about number of operatories, however; it's also how you use them, schedule them, and turn them over efficiently. Happiness for a dentist is each operatory full at eight AM. At least, that was Alex's definition when he owned the practice and had two associates working for him. Alex has a saying, "8 at 8." That meant he loved seeing eight cars in the patient parking lot as he pulled into work, four patients for the two dentists and four patients for the four hygienists to start each day.

Later, once Alex had sold his practice and was working more efficiently and only two days a week, he wanted 3-in-3: three patients in his three operatories at eight AM. One "A" appointment for big production, one "B" appointment for minor production, and one "C" appointment for his no production chair. For instance, that could be a crown, a filling, and an ortho check; or an endo, an extraction, and a crown seat. ABC, or as some call it, "Rock, Sand, Water."

Every dentist needs three to four operatories available to maximize effectiveness and efficiency. As time goes on, practices that have expanded to encompass multiple dentists in a single location with adequate number of operatories will be the most successful practices in town. They will also be the most valuable to buyers looking to purchase a dental practice.

The big take-away is: plan for your success. Think ahead and plan for the day you will want to add an associate dentist to your practice and the day you sell your practice. A minimum of five operatories and ideally, seven to ten, is a wise investment.

Alex thought, "My job just got a little easier with all those excellent answers showing up at the peck of a fingertip." Each dentist got an answer to a question to help them put another piece of their puzzle together. For Alex, happiness was each operatory full at eight AM. If you can figure out what makes you happy and starts your day well, you are half way to having a great day. Having what you need is how you build each day into a success.

The next time you have a question, consider the silicon sandbox and social networks, as well as Google and Wikipedia. LinkedIn and Facebook groups are like coffeehouses, where like-minded people gather to share ideas. There are hundreds of online dental groups where you can tap into the dental collective. Order a double macchiato and see who shows up. Start a group or join a group. Compare your Swiss Army knives and swap a few stories. The day is young, and you've a life to enjoy.

Chapter 13

FAMILY

Father Knows Best was a popular television show starring Robert Young and Jane Wyatt. It was filmed in black and white and depicted an idyllic American family, the Andersons. The parents, Jim and Margaret, were always wise and offered good, sound advice to their questioning offspring Bud, Betty, and Kathy.

Alex recommends that when you really want to know what's best, consider going back to your roots for answers. They'll usually have an objective answer guided by their interest in and close knowledge of your situation. They really do want what's best for you. That's why Alex referred the five protégés back to their families for input on their next set of questions.

FOLLOW-UP

Dr. Steve Blake's father had been in insurance sales, and when Steve asked him the key to success, he was quick to answer, "Follow-up." The fortune is in the follow-up.

Have you noticed that people on your team want to try to get people to make an appointment? This is not making cold calls. It is getting back in touch, following up with people who have expressed interest or been in for an exam and a consult, but have not yet started treatment.

Two types of patients need follow-up. (1) Those that responded to a marketing message but haven't come in for an exam, and (2) those that have had an exam, know they need treatment, but haven't gotten it yet. Most people think reactivating existing patients is the only follow-up needed, but what would happen if all those who shared your social media posts, liked your Facebook page, read your blog post, read your tweets, or reviewed YouTube videos about your practice were in a creative sales funnel for follow-up?

That would be an awesome follow-up system, especially if it were all automatic. That's a whole different level of follow-up from what you probably have right now. The good news is that it is being developed. Parts of the puzzle are already available and more is coming to further automate the process. Some of the software involves Maccrony, Ontraport, BleuPage, VideoBuilder, MSG Leads, Social Traffic Jacker, LiveCaster, StrikiVid, Liveleap, Conjurgram, Pushleads, Lead Shocker, WP Tweet Machine, Social Engage, and Mints Viral. Go to the resource list on Alex's website. Look for links to follow-up systems, dental software, and niche patient marketing ideas. Remember, the fortune is in the follow-up.

DECATHLON DENTISTRY

Dr. Blair Bennett's mother had four other children. Blair asked how she had chosen her dentist before Blair had graduated from dental school. She said that she chose a dentist where she could get everything done under one roof. She appreciated a comprehensively trained dentist.

Operating at maximum capacity means being able to perform every treatment your patient needs. That's being a decathlon dentist. Most dental graduates can do three or four procedures pretty well, and with experience perhaps five. To move up the capacity ladder, it is essential to continue your education as soon as possible.

Adding implants, sedation, TMD, and ortho to the mix will assure your ability to treat 90% of dental needs. The more you can do for one patient the more income you can create from the patients in your practice. Parents, usually the mother, tend to choose a dentist who can attend to the various needs of all their children, as did Dr. Bennett's mother.

The good hunter with many skills and a quiver full of arrows will kill the most meat, and you can't eat what you don't kill. A good number of dentists starve because they aren't "good hunters." They lack the skills or ability to perform certain tasks. It puts them at a disadvantage in the competitive arena.

One side note to being a decathlon dentist: You only need half the number of new patients as your non-decathlon competitors to produce the same amount of income. Looking at it another way, you can produce twice the income with the same number of new patients. Think about that. It should make a dentist think. Finally, another point: patients love going to a dentist who does it all. They like to get everything done under one roof. Many referrals, like prescriptions, go unfilled. When the patient can be served in your own facility by the people he or she already knows and trusts, everyone wins.

The decathlon dentist has been described as "beyond the average dentist." What about those who have incorporated alternative medical and dental training into their practices? Those are "holistic dentists," and that is another level of learning. Look into *The Holistic Dental Matrix*, by Dr. Nicholas Meyer. What we know and believe today is subject to change and revision as science catches up to reality.

WHAT'S ON YOUR WALLS?

Dr. Edward Boyle asked his wife for one key word of advice for his practice. She was a public relations executive for a Fortune 500 company and knew the value of getting a company's story out and keeping current customers informed. She said it was all about "the story." Social proof is huge in convincing potential patients to spend their health care dollars at your practice. Nowhere is it more important to show them than the walls of your office. What is on your walls? Do you have fine artwork, dental before and after photos, diplomas, certificates, patient testimonials, photos of mission trips, family, hobbies, or just ordinary prints? Do you utilize educational videos of dental products or procedures on oral health in your waiting room or operatories?

What's on your walls should tell a story. It should help the patient define you so that they bond to you and your practice. The team should go the extra mile during the new patient tour to explain the meaning of each piece of art, each honor, certificate, and personal photograph, as if they were the story board for a movie. Take time to construct your story and train your team to give tours that distinguish you from the competition. Engage the patient during the tour to get them to make the connection. How are they like you? How are they like the doctor? People prefer common ground as they begin to establish rapport and trust. This is the time and place to begin the bonding process.

NICHE FORMULA

Dr. Carley Matthews asked her uncle, the VP of sales at a successful local Internet marketing firm, "What is the best way to get high-quality patients? I need patients who want the kind of dentistry I'm trained to do." His job was to oversee the acquisition of new accounts, so he would know a lot about growth. If you want to attract high-end patients who want the specific type of dentistry you do, you need a customized marketing funnel to draw them in. I call that the niche-patient funnel formula.

Formula because it has parts that must fit into the equation, allowing it to work well.

Funnel because it takes the population of potential patients on the Internet, social media, and who listen to local radio and TV, and it draws in those who listen to the message that speaks to them.

Niche because it creates hoops potential patients must jump through to get into your office. The greater their desire to meet you, the greater your conversion rate or amount of dentistry completed will be. It's a screening process that provides the practice with quality, high-end, ready-to-buy patients.

High-end niche patient funnels are the future of dental marketing and perfect for a practice that is highly productive and able to accommodate new patients rapidly. How do you feed "the beast"? The $10,000-a-day dentist has a beast of a schedule. Wouldn't it be easier to schedule two or three nice-sized cases or one big case a day and not have to worry about engineering twenty patients into a crammed schedule?

That's where the niche patient funnel formula comes in. You market for specific types of high-end cases with a unique funnel formula, using imaginative, funny, and emotional ads on Facebook and Twitter. You use email, direct mail, contests, games, great offers, sterling headlines, outstanding follow-up, and strong calls to action. You dig to find the exact type patient you want. Imagine patients calling your practice who want a specific type of dental implant, like all-ceramic zirconia, a 360 smile makeover, the new 7-day Invisalign aligners, holistic ozone root canal treatment, All Under One Roof comprehensive dentistry, pearl veneers, or K7 neuromuscular TMD treatment. You know it's good when the best cases are calling you, not the competition. That's when you know your niche marketing funnel is working. That's how we feed the beast!

MULTITASKING

Dr. Jack Mudd lost his father at an early age, Alex learned during their talks. Over the years, they became close friends. Jack looked up to Alex even though they were relatively close in age. So Jack, when he needed fatherly advice, went to Alex. In answer to "What gave you the edge over other dentists? How were you able to be so consistently productive?" Alex said, "Being consistently productive is a skill and an art. You need the capacity to do it, the internal force that drives you to success. One element of that drive relates to your ability to multitask. In forty years of practice, I've worked with over twenty associate dentists. I've seen them work, heard them talk, and studied their schedules. I've tried to teach them all to be more efficient and work smarter, not harder. There is a lot to be learned from observing other dentists. What I found was that some dentists just have more capacity than other dentists to produce. A lot of it comes from mindset, attitude, and their ability to multitask.

"Multitasking means you can think on two or three levels at once. You can think in parallel, not just serially. Preparing a crown prep in Operatory A doesn't take all your energy. You are equally comfortable having a new patient being toured by your team, a crown being tried in Operatory B, and an ortho wire change in Operatory C. When two hygienists lay their route cards behind you on the counter, you do mental gymnastics of when to stop your current procedure and check their patients. A dentist that can multitask will not collapse under this type of pressure. A dental practice with efficient systems will enable a multitasker to operate at a significantly higher level of productivity than the average practice. When you are the master of your emotions and the strong director of a team in whom you are confident, you have a high capacity for success."

Chapter 14

BRINGING PRAYER TO BEAR

Prayer is essential for a successful practice and life. Connecting to the creator will give you insights and inspiration to go further, do better, and be at greater peace than any other method. Many in the business world want to avoid this approach, but I feel just the opposite. I believe the primary reason we have been doubly blessed (Job 42:12 and Isaiah 61:7-9) is because we prayed for guidance and revelation, received it, and acted on it in faith. I urge you to buck the current politically correct system and put prayer back to work in and for your business, your life, and your family. The fruit you will see will be abundant (Job 42:10 and Zechariah 9:12).

Alex spent forty-seven years trying to do things his way. It was only after turning everything over to God and praying for direction that the struggle left and the path became clear. "Clarity comes to the one willing to do the will of God," said Bill Johnson. Alex grew his practice to nearly six million in just ten years. Listening to that still, small voice became a habit he never forgot. Nearly twenty years later, Alex still counsels those who have ears to hear. Alex advised his five protégés to find their quiet places and meditate in prayer, speak their fears, their desires, their adoration, and their joy to the One who is above all. Then he advised them to be still and listen. It's in the listening that one connects to greater wisdom and insights are seen and understood.

Alex routinely asked each of his students what they were hearing. He was interested in where the Lord would lead them and how that might impact their future decisions. These are the revelations they shared.

TEAM CAPABILITY AND DELEGATION

Dr. Jack Mudd received a revelation on the value of involving his team more, continuing a theme that the team is the key to breaking free. Jack yearned to be free and saw where this fit into the plan for his practice.

"The ideal mindset of a $10,000-a-day dentist," said Alex, "is that your team is capable, can do everything well, and take care of patients exquisitely. All duties that are delegable, they can do."

When Alex was in dental school at the Medical College of Georgia, three of the classes he took were DAU (Dental Auxiliary Utilization) EDAU (Expanded Duty Auxiliary Utilization), and TEAM = (Training in Expanded Auxiliary Management). In these classes, he learned to think and work productively. Don't waste time doing it yourself if you can delegate it to a prepared and effective member of the team. Training is the key.

"Whatever your two hands can do, four can do better. What happens in Operatories 2 and 3 can be amazingly productive while you are working in Room 1. If hands are income centers, doesn't it make sense to maximize the opportunity per operatory? Your team is capable and delegation is desirable."

EXPERT STATUS

Dr. Carley Matthews saw the light shining on the hill and knew it was meant for her. She saw her name in lights. She saw herself as others did, as the expert in complex dentistry. She and Alex had this conversation about her answers to prayer.

What are those initials after your name and what do they have to do with your success?

The patient's perception makes the difference as to whom they choose for their dentist, so we should all strive to be seen in the best light possible. The dentist most patients want to see is the expert in their craft. You have a distinct advantage over your competition if you are seen as the local expert. An expert has more training, higher education, better equipment, greater skill, a stronger team, and superior results. Why wouldn't a potential patient prefer the expert?

Patients find the expert because someone lets them know who they are, where they are, and when they can be seen. Are you letting the public know everything they need to know about your expert status?

Are you seen as the authority in your town?

INTERVIEW ROOM

Dr. Blair Bennett received confirmation to her prayer. She needed an extravagant place to connect with her patients and establish rapport since she was a new dentist. Alex showed her how her answered prayer would have an impact on how she would build the trust needed to become her patients' dentist for a lifetime.

Alex explained that the extravagance of an interview room, a second consult room, to meet and greet your new patients would catapult her practice. In a busy practice, the patient treatment coordinator is going to be using her consult room

50-75% of the day, if not more. That means you need a free space, away from dental therapy operatories, to interview your new patients.

The interview room is a key part of the new patient experience, a place to sit knee-to-knee with new patients to establish rapport in a non-dental environment and gain understanding of why they are there. Alex likes to use this room for his interviews because it's not a threatening environment, it frees up operatories for productive dentistry, and it helps manage the flow of patients better. It's a holding tank, if you will, allowing the dentist to plan interactions with the new patient more professionally.

In the interview room, the new patient coordinator goes over the medical and dental history, smile evaluation forms, and the patient's "story." Once the story is known, the team tunes the doctor in to the patient's wishes. The transfer of this vital information occurs in two places: outside the interview room privately with the dentist and inside again in the presence of the patient so that they know that their story and needs have been heard and transferred to the doctor by the team.

Remember, everything is scripted, and at every turn there are specific lines and events. The interview room is one set on the stage of a three-part play. As we tour our patients during the new patient experience, they are the audience; they are the ones to whom we deliver our lines. Team members who know their lines and how to hit the mark when called upon are the most valuable team members.

SCHEDULE TO GOAL – ABC

God answered Dr. Steve Blake with a finite strategy of utmost elegance: scheduling to goal. This turned out to be one of the most important lessons Steve ever got. It contained the Wisdom of Solomon. God is good! When Steve and Alex discussed the revelation Steve received, Alex explained what it meant.

The most important factor in being a $10,000-a-day dentist is having your team schedule to your goal. Without that primary mindset, your results will be inconsistent, like target practice without a target. Without an objective or production goal to aim for, your scheduling team could easily miss your goal. Once the ground work of a strong daily goal is laid, the parts are added to make it an easy and consistent reality.

Engineering the perfect day schedule is the job of the doctor's appointment secretary. Keeping the schedule full and productive is a necessary function of the team, however. Our Humpty Dumpty schedule falls off the wall at times and we need to be experts at putting Humpty Dumpty back together again. Hygienists, clinical assistants, dentists, and business assistants play a role in the construction and maintenance of the $10,000-a-day schedule. Alex recommends the ABC approach for scheduling:

> "A" for rock, or big item dentistry in column one,
> "B" for sand, or small treatment items in column two, and the
> "C" column is for water or no dollar production dental visits.

Alex also recommends an extra operatory for conversions, overflow, and emergency work-ins. Keep it filled every day, employ well-trained, cross-trained teams of clinical assistants for delegated duties, and learn to say Yes as often as you can to patients' needs and requests.

Starting with the end in mind, $10,000 per day, you will soon be reaching your goal on a consistent basis.

REPUTATION

Dr. Edward Boyle was to be a featured worker in the Kingdom. God gave Edward a peek at how a true servant should tell his story. The message: "People love to go to a dentist who has the reputation of being a giver."

Alex enjoyed hearing this and relayed his own story about building a desirable reputation. Success comes from telling your story well. Engage people with your story, and they will like you. Entertain people, and they will share your story. These are the steps to gaining first a foothold and then creating a viral explosion of positive impressions about you and your practice. When you have a good story to tell, don't keep it a secret. Remember the TV detective drama *The Naked City*? Its closing line was, "There are eight million stories in the naked city. This has been one of them." A dental practice has hundreds of stories to tell. A mission-minded dentist, like Dr. Boyle, will have thousands of heart-warming stories to share. Share the grand stories of your travels, your family, and your missions. Make your patients feel like they are with you and your team on your mission journeys. When you can vicariously take your patients on a journey with you to the wilds of the African Masai Mara you create a link, a bond that will remain strong and unbroken.

Then Alex dove deeper into how dentists use the media to get their message out to those who are and would become patients in their practices. "What's changed since we first built our five million-dollar practice? Social media and mobile devices overtook the web. When I began to pay attention to getting online reviews on my web site, I began to average over $10,000 a day. If you combine good stories with great reviews, you get an avalanche of new patients."

Alex believes there is a direct correlation between your online reputation and the caliber of patients you attract to your practice. Think of your few poor online reviews as a giant cyber screen where the only patients who get through are those not negatively affected by bad reviews. Consider your wonderful pool of great reviews as a huge magnetic funnel that sweeps many patients into your practice. The type of patients who respond to good stories and great reviews will have high trust and loyalty to your practice. They are worth gold to you and your future.

An excellent reputation is hard to achieve and easy to lose. Develop a plan to monitor and protect your reputation. A proactive stance is the key to reputation management. Now that social media and mobile access to information reigns, be sure your reputation is front and center. Keep it a daily focus.

Alex's Personal Story: Bringing God Back into the Work Place

Alex received the anointing of the Holy Spirit as an adult. He was pleased to see that his protégés had heard from God and understood as they had listened. The words they had received were on target and just what they needed to hear at that moment in their careers. God's timing is always perfect, thought Alex. He smiled as he remembered his calling, to bring God back into the workplace. That was the word he received in 1997. He got a second chance to get it right and he tried to leave that message with those who had ears to hear. The anointing is given to enhance what one is gifted to do.

"Nothing is more powerful than an anointed professional on their job."

Pastor Jentezen Franklin

How often have you heard that a particular doctor's hands are anointed, that they have a gift for a particular procedure? What if not only one's hands were anointed but also their speech, their vision, their understanding, and their compassion? The Spirit regularly provides fresh, creative insight to those who are well-grounded and have an open mind. That is precisely how Alex received his two goals, his daily goal and his eight AM goal, to teach his fellow dentists to be successful.

An anointed person is able to do things ordinary people cannot do. Prayer can reshape one's career, life, and family.

Prayer is the place to seek answers that no one else can answer. Connecting to the Creator of all the universe and receiving guidance gives a person peace that surpasses all understanding. It's true that God answers prayers and can even help shape one's day…every day.

A Confession

Does Alex seem very familiar to the author—his inner thoughts and attitudes? Yes, Alex is just my pen name, my alter ego. I wanted my readers to put themselves under the tutelage of a mentor and take a journey that would dramatically impact their lives. I'm sure my friends who know me figured it out early and were going to ask the question as soon as they read through the illustrations. I just thought I'd just admit it here and save them the call!

In my earlier book, *Marketing the Million Dollar Practice*, the chapter "The Prayer of Jabez" detailed how I found that book and how meaningful it was to us in our early days. I prayed daily for many months, and it became a habit to continue to be in prayer for our family and our practice. Such is the real-time power of prayer. Indeed, the three-ply strand of hearing, believing, and faith has given me a peace and balance that was missing in my early days. As time and events passed, I changed, and the nature of my prayers also changed. I'd like to share one such prayer that I still use to start my day. I call it my "parking lot" prayer.

My Morning Parking Lot Prayer

Lord, thank you for all of your blessings for my practice, Suwanee Dental Care, for our team members, and for our wonderful patients. May all our treatments, examinations, and diagnoses be correct today and be guided by your hand. Lord, I pray for provision for our practice, our team and for each patient to have the financial ability to afford the dentistry they need. I declare that Suwanee Dental Care is a $6,300,000 production *and collection practice for 2017 and pray that we meet and exceed our goals. In Jesus's name, Amen.*

And do you know what? God answered our prayers year after year. We always had enough to do what we needed, go where we wanted to, and serve as we were led to serve. We achieved our goals and more, always in abundance. Do you also have a morning parking lot prayer?

Speaking of praying for outcomes, I have one more outcome I want to share with you. We are near the end of this book, and we have traveled a path together, along with Alex and his five dentist friends. I'm not sure you knew where we were headed or what to expect, but that's why it's called a journey. I'm glad we could do it together. My wish now is that you find success and happiness through your life's work. I pray for an outstanding outcome for you and your family.

This Is My Prayer for You

Lord, I thank you for sending this excellent person to me through this book. I see that you have opened a window for them to view into the heavenly realm and to imagine the possibilities of what you have in store for them in their future. I pray that they will maintain access to you and your goodness and that you will bestow upon them health, wealth, and wisdom. I pray that you bring into their life people of faith and wisdom who will walk beside them and help them navigate the alleyways of life. Lord, I pray that you will speak to them and give them guidance when they ask. In Jesus's name, Amen.

Chapter 15

STICK TO IT: DON'T GET OFF THE TRAIN

The Alvia Euro Express train from Madrid pulled out on time, as it always did. It was late afternoon, nearly five PM, and the Spanish family of five who had adopted me for the day and fed me a lovely meal of paella and Sangria now waved adios from the train platform, tears trickling down the young nina's cheeks because the American, her new friend, was leaving so soon. I was on the move again: destination Pamplona, the home of the running of the bulls.

Three hours and three minutes later, my train pulled into Pamplona. The skies were darkened and it was raining a torrent from the solid bank of steel grey clouds. I made an instant decision to stay onboard the Alvia using my Eurail Pass and ride northward. The train was Paris bound and why not? I could sleep on the train and arrive the next morning in the City of Lights. By the time I arrived at Gare du Nord, the sky was a pale blue, morning rays escaping over the horizon illuminating the Eiffel Tower on the cityscape. I was rested for another day of adventure along the Champs Elysees.

That was one day on my backpacking tour of Europe via the Eurail system back in 1972, after completing my college degree at Auburn University before beginning dental studies at the Medical College of Georgia. I had a plan to see all of Europe in ten weeks, starting in London. I had my itinerary and transportation all lined up. All I needed to do was be at Heathrow airport at the end of the ten weeks to return home. Where I went in between and when was totally up to me to decide. All I had to do was stick to the plan.

The Eurail pass was a godsend when I didn't know where I wanted to go until the last minute. The options were always there. I could hop aboard any train, ride first-class. It was like a free pass to anywhere. Many times over the ten-week excursion I found that it was good to have unlimited options, especially when it was raining and I didn't want to get wet!

When you have freedom to roam, to do what you want, life can be so much more enjoyable. There is a time to work, and a time to play, and a time to rest. Balancing the Cross of Life never goes out of style. I wanted to show the reader that it is possible to work hard and store enough money so that when the time comes, you have unlimited choices on how you want to live. I want everyone to be able to "finish well." But to do that, you sometimes have to make the decision to stay on the train.

Do You Have The Right Tools?

We all need tools to navigate life. The Eurail pass is a good example. You gain spontaneity when you have the right tools. For a dentist who is chained to the chair with golden handcuffs, feeling that he or she cannot escape for fear of loss of income, the overhead monster, and critical patient care, I recommend the following:

1. This book's fifty ways to become a $10,000-a-day dentist,

2. The 5M Masters Academy and its fifteen online modules on how to create a five million dollar practice, and
3. The 5M Mastermind where one doctor sharpens another.
4. Create an investment portfolio that will grow and allow you to do what you want to do once you decide it is time to slow down and eventually retire.

These are all tools on your Swiss Army knife, tools to inspire excellence in your work and enable you to carve out a little rest, relaxation, and fun in your life. My theory has always been that the dentist who plans and prepares well then works hard with perseverance will have a rewarding career and enjoyable retirement. Work enough hours when young so you can work fewer hours when you are older. I firmly believe in the four-day work week after one is out of debt from school loans. Work five, even six, days a week until that day. Stick to your budget and stay out of debt. Save more than you spend and invest in secure, not flashy, investments. Work now; play later.

Those who apply the Swiss Army knife principles to dentistry will be able to slow down as they reach the mature stage of their practice. Those will indeed be the golden years of their careers. They'll have more time and money to travel as they wish. Taking cruises on the Danube, ski trips to Whistler, a villa in Cancun, renting a condo in Maui for a month, or exploring the ancient cobblestone streets of Prague will all be an option if one plans well to finish well.

POINTS TO PONDER—REFLECTING BACK

The road to success is paved with many stones, each laid by ones who've come before and blazed a trail, having done the hard work of clearing the jungle. This book tells the story of Alex, who traveled the trail early and often, who knows the nuances of the game of dentistry, and who passes on his accumulated wisdom to those that would follow.

Above all else, Alex desires that each dentist be successful in the realm of his or her own desire. He wants each professional to feel alive and have a fire burning in their hearts for their patients, team, and family. As not everyone wants success in the same measure, this book is designed to encourage dentists to define success in a way that fits their image of a good life. Seeking balance is as important as seeking practice growth and profits. Seeking God is just as important as finding family time and fulfilling vacations. Dentistry is a profession, not a life. Alex implores all dentists to get a life before they get too old to enjoy it.

When I first founded Solstice Dental Advisors, my consulting firm for dentists, I created a logo with four different colored leaves. They represent the four seasons of the year and the four seasons of a dentist's life. Only a dentist in his or her fourth season can understand the life cycle of a dentist fully, and it has been my passion to try and share this by representing each of the four seasons in this book by introducing you to Blaire, Edward, Carley, and Steve. It's not hard to understand how following Alex's recommendations will enable each of them to finish well.

That leaves Jack. Jack represents all those who are not initially growers, seekers, or even open-minded, and there are a lot of those in dentistry. I wanted this book to be for all dentists, so it had to include Jack, who had a coming out party during his time in the dental hot seat with Alex. Perhaps the greatest value of this book could be that many dentists whose fires are but embers could somehow catch flame with this renewing fuel.

Where to go from here?

If you want to read more, Dr. Williams' *Marketing the Million Dollar Practice* is available on Amazon. He has also collaborated on and published his edition of *Smile 360: A Patient's Guide to Cosmetic Dentistry*. To join the 5M Masters Online Academy or the next available 5M Mastermind, go to the websites sited and signup or request additional information. Those who participate in these forums will experience the best of what Dr. Williams has to offer.

Quotes from Members of the 5M Mastermind

Mark Braydich, Braydich Dental in Hubbard, Ohio:

- "Work with Bill at Solstice Dental Advisors because he is the real deal. He's honest, straightforward, and experienced. He's done everything that he's trying to teach you. The return on your investment will be threefold."

- "Bill is an open book. He is willing to help and work with anybody. You could call him at any time, any day, email. He was there for you. He gets you focused. He talks about $10,000 a day, which is a pretty outstanding goal, and he talks about the ways to achieve that and make it fun."

- "A lot of times you'll go and see a speaker and they aren't actually in there doing it. He's been practicing and he's doing it. He could really relate to you about the good and the bad. He really helped us with scheduling and it was able to increase our productivity. Things are running smoother and that was a really big boost to our practice."

- "He has a ton of online content. It'll take a long time to go through all of that. But if you do get through all of it, you're going to be much more productive. Not only for the dentist but also for their staff."

Brad Hester, Bend Family Dentistry in Bend, Oregon:

- "Work with Solstice Dental Advisers because your results will amaze you. Money very well spent. Bill, he's a really sharp, sharp, sharp dentist and businessman. I have always been a fairly big number producer but he helped us institute hitting $10,000 a day consistently and continue to do so. There's no question that Bill Williams is a teacher that can provide results to your practice and your everyday life."

- "You want to get the team involved with your process and your goal of $10,000 a day and make it fun for them so that you can all celebrate together. That really makes a difference."

- "The friendships that I have made in the Mastermind group are lifetime. Bill and I still communicate and he still gives input to me. We stay connected."

Gregg May, Deep South Family Dentistry in Ponchatoula, Louisiana:

- "Work with Solstice Dental Advisors because it's worth every penny. The ROI on working with Bill will always be tenfold from what you think the investment is in the beginning."

- "Bill is a very well respected, very talented individual who has learned from some of the best masters in our profession. He has so much to share and so much to offer the general community as a whole. Everyone should take some time to get to know Bill and listen to some things that he has to say."

- "Bill has been a success. A young dentist or a new dentist or even an older dentist sometimes doesn't realize their potential. And a $10,000 day is much easier to achieve with systems in place and protocols in place and mentoring that's easily available through Bill. He has put everything he's learned into other people."

Dr. Kevin Poupore in Malone, New York:

- "Work with Solstice Dental Advisors because Dr. Bill, he's the real deal. He's not some pie in the sky guy. I just can't recommend them enough. On a 5-star rating system I give them 10. The camaraderie is tremendous. He looks at your exact situation, he helps you fix whatever's wrong. It's worth the investment."

- "He has modules that you can use online to learn certain areas. What I get the most out of is when I go right to his home and we're part of a mastermind group. You'll sit in front of everybody and explain how you're doing. Then he'll help you diagnose what you can do differently to make it better. He has a concept on being a $10,000 a day dentist. Now I'm a $15,000 a day dentist, just from getting the idea from him and all the little nuts and bolts and how to implement it."

- "He wants you to improve other parts of your life as well as just being a dentist. He doesn't just focus in on the practice, he tries to help you see that you need to read other things; you need to be paying attention to your family and your health. We talk about that in a mastermind group."

- "He wants you to get out in the community and help other people to do what they're interested in as well. It's like a cycle. You help other people, they help you. It's important in any aspect of your life to do what you believe."

- "At the end of each mastermind session he gives you a prescription for what you want to work on. Of course, when you go back, they ask you how did you do. The same with once a month mastermind phone call and then people ask you, 'Well, how did you do on what you wanted to accomplish?'"

- "I'm in his mastermind group. I've done it now two years and I just love it. I live in a rural area and I like to be around other high-level, high-performing dentists. Dr. Williams is like the guru's guru. He knows everything there is to know about dentistry and marketing. He tweaks everybody to help them maximize their performance. He wants you to rev up and do even better. He's fantastic."

Rudy Braydich of Braydich Dental in Hubbard, Ohio:

- "We took a leap of faith and joined up with Dr. Bill and we have not been disappointed. One of the great things, the mastermind group met at his home every quarter and we're able to have individual one-on-one time with Bill which was priceless. Considering the cost of the course and the fact that you have one-on-one time with the instructor, it's just awesome."

- "The amount of money that you're putting in it is significant, but when you see the amount of time that you get to spend with one of the more successful dentists in the country and the other connections that you make, it's priceless."

- "Relationships are very important and Bill is very concerned about making sure that he has good relationships with doctors that he's working with. He introduced us to a lot of different techniques that they're using in his dental practice. He understands what's going on on a day-to-day basis, today, not five years ago. He's able to bring different techniques and different suggestions and improve our work environment and hit the goals that we wanted."

- "Bill leads by example, I think that's one of the greatest attributes that he has. He shows his own statistics of how he used the same idea and what it did for him. One of the things that my brother and I love doing is copying off of successful people. It's better than trying to recreate the wheel and Bill was willing to open up and show us everything that he was doing to become successful. We just latched on to that and it has done great rewards for us. Our practice was leveling off, $3.5 million. Last year we did $4.1. This year we're looking at doing $5."

- "His marketing strategies are awesome. I'm in a little community of 15,000 people and we're the big fish in a little pond because we use the principles that he uses. There's some things that never change if you decide to engage in those principles. We're one of the best dental practice in our area."

- "Bill is a very, very detailed person and he has every "I" dotted and every "T" crossed in every type of system that you can possibly think of. There are many times when we all hit $10,000 a day which is very exciting. Our staff now is crystal clear on that vision and it's all through the teachings. You have to experience it to understand it but you won't be disappointed."

RESOURCES

Everyone needs an "Alex" in their life. Can you do it by yourself? Sure, but that's the definition of a silo dentist, one who is isolated and goes it alone, one who lives behind the walled city and does not mix and match with others. Find your "Alex" and study the path they took. Don't hesitate to seek guidance because the Guide will keep you from stepping into the quicksand in the dental jungle. Only the Guide can give you the Swiss Army knife you need to institute strategies like the Gold Key List, the Leap Frog Strategy, and more.

How to Connect with "Alex":

Request a consultation:
http://SolsticeDentalAdvisors.com/Mastermind

1. **Order the Books**: *Marketing the Million Dollar Practice*, by Dr. Bill Williams
https://www.amazon.com/Marketing-Million-Dollar-Practice-Williams/dp/1619200120
Smile 360: A Patient's Guide to Cosmetic Dentistry by Dr. Bill Williams. Order the Book at https://goo.gl/CMoj5B at MagCloud.com

2. **Join the online 5M Masters Academy**: http://solsticedentaladvisors.com/5macademy
3. **Apply for the next 5M Mastermind:** http://solsticedentaladvisors.com/mastermind/
4. **Connect on Social Media:**
   Facebook - https://www.facebook.com/SolsticeDentalAdvisors/
   LinkedIn - https://www.linkedin.com/in/billwilliamsdmd
   Twitter - https://twitter.com/wbwilliams
   Pinterest - https://www.pinterest.com/drbillwilliams/

Appendix 1:

DEFINITIONS

3 in 3: Having three patients booked for three operatories for an A, B, and C procedure, respectively. Generally for one dentist at eight AM.

5M: The Five Million-Dollar Practice, defined by the online 5M Masters Academy and the live 5M Mastermind training sessions, by Dr. Bill Williams.

8@8: Seeing eight automobiles in the parking lot at eight AM representing eight patients booked for eight operatories at the dental practice

Dental hot seat: A mastermind strategy that places a dentist and his or her practice in the spotlight to dissect the present situation, define the obstacles, and suggest a prescription for resolution of problem areas.

Extra dental perception: Study and application of business principles from outside the traditional dental practice approach.

Free time anytime: Having the financial and schedule freedom to come and go, be it work or vacation, as one wishes.

Funnel analysis: Funnel analysis involves using a series of events that lead towards a defined goal, like from patient engagement in a mobile app, to an NPE, on to acceptance of treatment at the consult, and completing a crown appointment a few weeks later. The funnel analyses are effective ways to calculate conversion rates on specific patient behaviors in the form of a purchase, multiple purchases, or other intended actions from patients.

Gap analysis: A system utilized to determine which steps should to be taken in order to move from its current state to its desired state. Also called need-gap analysis, needs analysis, and needs assessment. It includes (1) listing of characteristic factors, such as attributes, competencies, and performance levels of the present situation – what is, (2) listing factors needed to achieve future objectives – what should be, and then (3) highlighting the gaps, often as a percentage, that exist and need to be filled.

Gold key list: A chronological list of steps to take to advance from zero to a multimillion-dollar practice.

KPI: Key performance indicators are measurements of important elements of practice numbers, processes, and activities that are tracked over time to enable analysis of success or failure.

Leap frog strategy: Improving on systems and strategies in existence with innovative additions to surpass your competition.

Niche patient funnel formula: Marketing to a specific type patient for niche services like implants, Invisalign, cosmetic makeovers, veneers, All-on-Four Hybrid Dentures, and such, with specific marketing approaches that involve data mining, social media, mailing lists, educational materials, in-office presentations to the public, and follow-up.

NPE: New patient experience, as practiced and taught by Dr. Bill Williams for the past thirty years, where the tour of the practice occurs before the tour of the mouth.

Swiss Army knife approach: A combination of having a multitude of skills, à la the decathlon dentist, to handle any task at hand and the mindset and capacity to overcome any obstacle.

The 100-Day Challenge: Following Dr. Bill Williams through his one hundred video blog days living life, doing dentistry, challenging viewers, training clients, traveling abroad, and being with family and friends.

The Austrian thing: Enjoying conversation with friends in a coffee house.

The Dental Jungle: A series of LinkedIn articles by Dr. Bill Williams following Alex the Guide as he introduces his five dentists to ways to successfully navigate the untamed and often-times wild dental jungle.

The Red iPad: A method using an iPad chairside in the dental office to gain patients' agreement to place reviews and testimonials on online review sites. Links are sent to the patient's email address for proper IP address location.

The Trump Effect: Achieving surprising or unexpected positive results in economic indicators and outcomes by applying improved listening focus, innovative business management principles, and sticking to proven core values.

Appendix 2:

50 WAYS TO BECOME A $10,000-A-DAY DENTIST

Sorted and listed below are the individual recommendations that Alex made to the dentists as to which of "The Big Five" they most support. By studying each of the ten segments, the reader will be able to more successfully integrate the ideas and concepts that create the focus and change needed to have a consistently productive dental practice. For further growth, the team could elect to take each of the five segments and work to incorporate the ideas, i.e., Mindset, fully into their practice before moving to the next segment, i.e., Team, and so on.

1. Mindset

100% Readiness Chapter 4	Page 31
Advance Planning Chapter 5	Page 34
Fees, Financing, and Family Focus Chapter 5	Page 36
Comprehensive Dentistry Chapter 6	Page 40
Same Day Dentistry – Say Yes Chapter 6	Page 41
Goals and Results Chapter 7	Page 48
100% Willingness – Great Attitude Chapter 9	Page 66
Patient-Focus – Not Self-Focus Chapter 9	Page 70
KPI and The Gold Key List Chapter 11	Page 85
Team Capability and Delegation Chapter 14	Page 114

2. Team

3. Facility

4. Marketing

5. Capacity

Appendix 3:

GOLD KEY LIST

(Referenced in Chapter 2)

Many of the individual items on the Gold Key List are taught, instructed, explained, workshopped, and written about in the 5M Masters Online Academy, the 5M Mastermind, and the three Solstice Dental Practice Manuals (Business Assistants Manual, Dental Assistants Manual, and Dental Hygiene Manual). These resources are available for purchase by dentists and teams who wish to engage in a hands-on, growth-oriented practice refinement.

Gold Key List

1. Study visions & mission statements of other businesses and dental practices to get ideas for your own.
2. Plan Rock Time to get away for planning.
3. Create vision with your spouse.
4. Review vision with your key players.
5. Share vision with the team.
6. Publish vision – Frame and put in reception area.
7. Create the mission with your team.
8. Publish the mission.
9. Create culture points.

10. Publish culture points along with vision & mission on the website, office manuals, etc.
11. Develop a strategic plan for your practice.
12. Set goals for 5 years.
13. Set goals for 4 years.
14. Set goals for 3 years.
15. Set goals for 2 years.
16. Set goals for one year.
17. Do a GAP analysis of your current treatment mix. What do you need to add?
18. Do a GAP analysis of your CE needs over the next few years.
19. Gather info on courses and make a plan to attend.
20. Determine if you need a mentor for this process.
21. Do a GAP analysis of your current facility.
22. Create your expansion plan goals.
23. Develop your leadership system (organizational chart).
24. Develop your management system for hiring & employee evaluation (i.e., Profile XT).
25. Develop a protocol for corrective action.
26. Develop your patient care systems. List and practice them for refinement.
    a. Realize that patient care involves much more than customer service.
    b. Efficiency, procedure mix, etc.
27. Plan how you will offer exceptional customer service.
28. Hold a staff meeting to discuss customer service. What are you already doing, what can you do better, and what can you add?
29. Start a patient reward system to encourage referrals, loyalty, longevity, big cases.
30. Create your performance evaluation to include six-month goal setting and career development, KPIs, and communication plans with your team.

31. Doctor develops ninety-day plan that is on target with the one-year goals.
32. Share your ninety-day plan with your team leaders and have them formulate department and personal ninety-day plans.
33. Team leaders share the ninety-day plan with other team members and have them create their individual ninety-day plans.
34. Outline your salary structure. How will you give raises related to performance evaluations?
35. Team leaders fill out their performance evaluations forms.
36. Doctor-conducted performance evaluation with each leader individually.
37. Team members complete their performance evaluations.
38. Team leaders conduct performance appraisals with each team member individually.
39. Start a staff reward system.
40. Stock and equip all ops the same for efficiency.
41. Plan to add the income centers once education has been completed.
42. Set up a plan to cross-train your team.
43. Set a time frame and begin to cross-train one team member.
44. Do a funnel analysis of how patients enter and flow through your practice.
45. GAP analysis of your need for new patients
46. Set goals for the number of needed new patients.
47. Design and write copy about practice and doctors for NP Packet.
48. Create your blueprint for the NPE.
49. Delegate implementation of the NPE to the team.

50. Introduce one new part of the packet and plan for the NPE each week until completed.
51. Put NPE in place ASAP.
52. Develop script for NP tour.
53. Role play tour at staff meetings.
54. Video and review tours being done as you practice and learn.
55. Write scripts for telephone.
56. Write scripts for how insurance is handled in your practice.
57. Write scripts on handling the NP phone calls.
58. Write scripts on handling a shopper call.
59. Write scripts for treatment protocols.
60. Write scripts for each department.
61. Stress the need for consistency on communication to patients throughout the office.
62. Review your consultation process.
63. Determine who will do case presentations.
64. Select a marketing coordinator on your team to facilitate projects.
65. Do a GAP analysis of your marketing efforts.
66. Determine your marketing budget.
67. Determine your media mix and what you need to add.
68. Develop a MAP – marketing action plan for the short term.
69. Advertise your new procedures as you add them.
70. Evaluate website – does it need updating?
71. Add or update Facebook page, Twitter page, LinkedIn page.
72. Hire a company to assist you or make a team member accountable to manage social media.
73. Delegate to the team the parts of social media content and creation that they can do. Make it fun!

74. Select a group of external marketing resources that you will put into play over the next year.
75. Get all clinical staff on the expanded duty track ASAP.
76. Set up Google calendar for the doctors.
77. Set up Google calendar for the practice.
78. Set up Google documents for your seminar notes, staff meeting notes, etc.
79. Review each Solstice 5M module with your team.
80. Use staff meeting to formulate goals and action plans for each module.
81. Join a dental study club or create one if there isn't an active one in your area.
82. Place certificates, diplomas, and other interesting artifacts on the walls.
83. Implement the Red iPad.
84. Put patient testimonials online, in print, or on the air.
85. Choose a mentor to assist you each step of the way.
86. Identify and evaluate all systems currently in use in your practice.
87. Compare them to the Solstice systems and determine any tweaking that you want to do.
88. Have a team discussion on systems that work well.
89. Put your systems into a written form.
90. Implement a leadership training program.
91. Determine your insurance system:
    c. Do you verify insurance prior to patient's first visit?
    d. Do you update insurance at each visit or once a year?
    e. Do you accept insurance assignment?
    f. Do you participate in PPO programs?
92. Determine your collection system:
    a. Will you do any in-house financing?
    b. Set up patient financing option plan, i.e., Care Credit, LendingClub, Springstone.

   c. When do you call on overdue accounts?
   d. When do you send letters to overdue accounts?
   e. When do you turn accounts over to collections?
93. Develop or purchase an employee handbook with policies and procedures outlines.
94. Have each department record their systems and create department manuals for future training.
95. Employ efficiency techniques: delegate to your team.
96. Get input from your team on what is important to measure to understand the health of the practice.
97. Develop KPIs for your practice, individuals, and departments. Use the samples on the Solstice website to assist you.
98. Compile KPI scorecards into one form for doctor to evaluate.
99. Review and discuss KPI practice scorecard at doctor meetings, staff meeting, etc. Make it a useful topic of discussion to improve the practice.
100. Review your success in each of the Gold Key points and rework any points that are in need of updating.

ABOUT THE AUTHOR

William B. Williams, DMD, a recognized authority in general dentistry, dental implants, head, neck, and facial pain, marketing and dental practice management for forty-two years, is the author of *Marketing the Million Dollar Practice* and *Smile 360: A Patient's Guide to Cosmetic Dentistry*. He is the founder of Suwanee Dental Care and Solstice Dental Advisors, where he currently lives and works in Suwanee, Georgia. He and his wife Sheila are the proud parents of Will and Tyler and enjoy visiting Will, their daughter-in-law, Sarah, and granddaughter, Harper, in the United Kingdom.

ACKNOWLEDGMENTS

I would like to take a moment to convey my sincerest thanks and appreciation to some very special people who have contributed to my success, particularly as it relates to this, my most recent book. I'm thankful to God for life, Jesus for being my friend, and the Holy Spirit for giving me insights and inspiration when I ask.

To my life partner, my wife Sheila, who also shares in creating the works we do as chief practice management consultant for Solstice Dental Advisors in charge of practice development, manual preparation, is chief financial officer, and of course, keeper of feet on the ground for all my wild ideas!

I wish to acknowledge my son Tyler Williams for working with me in the Solstice business and particularly in the presentation of the 5M Mastermind and 5M Masters Academy online program as we developed the websites, funnels, webinars, and marketing for the courses. He has been an active contributor, a coach, a presenter, a marketing advisor, a copywriter, and much more.

I would like to thank Susan Hess for editing my manuscript multiple times after I edited a copy from an earlier time. She has been my executive assistant in Solstice Dental Advisors over the past two years, helping to keep me on track.

To my publisher, Deborah Greenspan, and editor, Bonnie Cox, at Breezeway Books who took a good look at my penned work and perfected it into a much more readable manuscript.

To you, I say, "Nice work!" I also want to thank Shari Reimann, the book designer at Breezeway, who turned that manuscript into an actual book that I can share with you.

To my office manager, sister-in-law, and Solstice consultant, Angie Cain, who has been a loyal helper and supporter, and a contributor to my teaching and coaching businesses for decades. She is the glue in my office and a respected coach and consultant to dentists.

To my many talented dentists, dental assistants, dental hygienists, lab technicians, business assistants, co-workers, and employees over the years at Stone Mountain Dental Group, Suwanee Dental Care, and Solstice Dental Advisors, who are too numerous to name but who know that they were and remain a vital part of my success as a dentist.

Ultimately none of this could have been done without the loyalty and support of our tens of thousands of patients over forty-two years. You believed in me and you allowed me to be your dentist. For that, I am honored.

Finally to all my colleagues in dentistry, particularly the original Solstice Group (Joe Ellis, Lee Ostler, Tommy Oppenheim, John Willoughby, Geoff Pratt, Tony Roeder, Steve Cobble, and Nick Meyer), who showed me a better way and positively impacted my life while giving me hope that there was a brighter future waiting at the end of the journey.

Thanks to all. You made this book possible with your years of service and encouragement to share what I know with my profession.

INDEX

B

C

D

E

F

G

H

I

J

K

L

M

N

O

P

Q

R

S

T

U

V

W

Y

Z

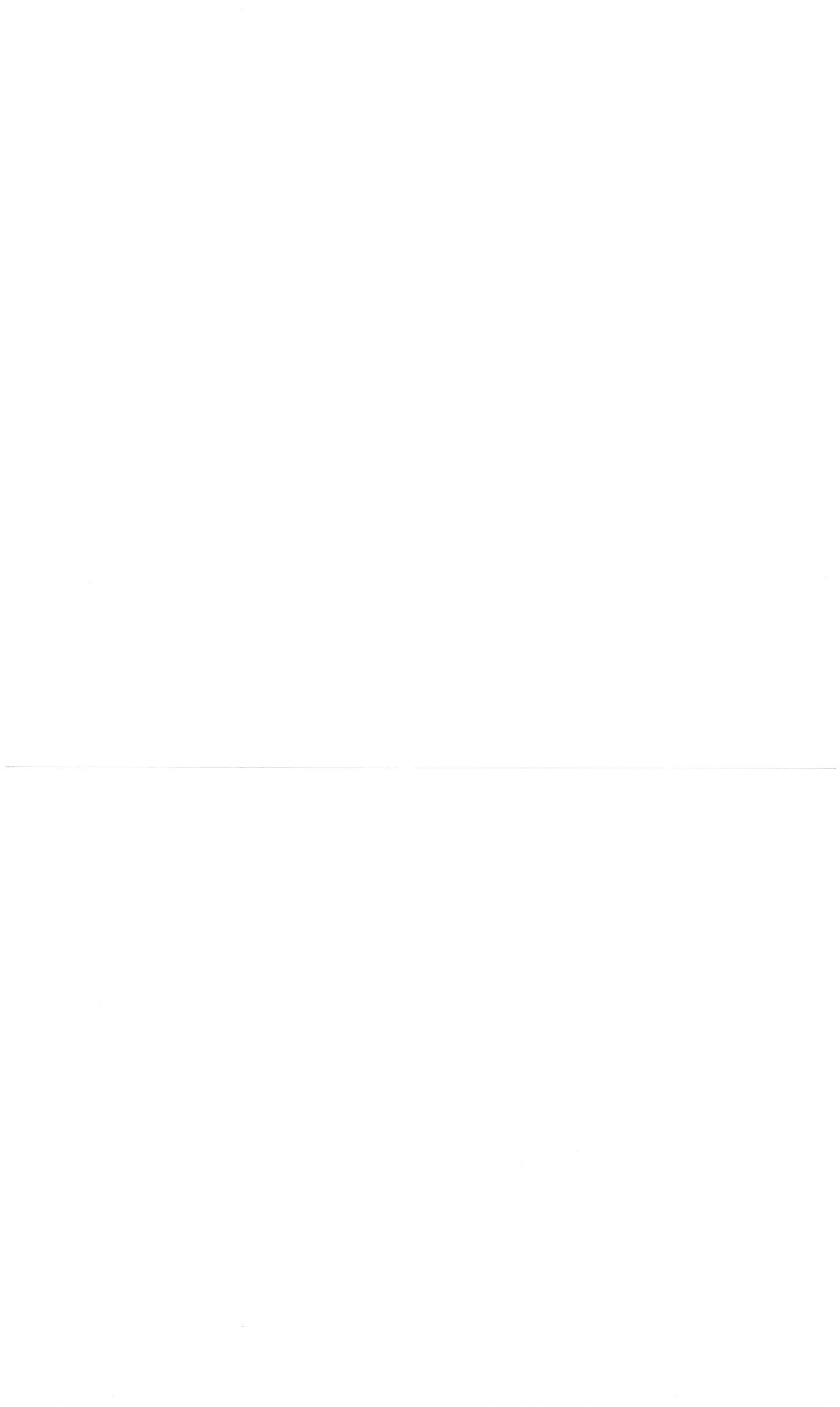

59326323R00106

Made in the USA
Middletown, DE
10 August 2019